# MENOPAUSE

## ALL YOUR QUESTIONS ANSWERED

## RAYMOND G. BURNETT, M.D.

CONTEMPORARY
BOOKS, INC.
CHICAGO ▪ NEW YORK

**Library of Congress Cataloging-in-Publication Data**

Burnett, Raymond, 1936–
    Menopause, all your questions answered.

    1. Menopause—Miscellanea.    2. Middle aged women—
Health and hygiene—Miscellanea.    I. Title. [DNLM:
1. Menopause—popular works.    WP    580    B964m]
RG186.B85        1987        618.1'75        87-19916
ISBN 0-8092-4677-5 (pbk.)

To my wife, Mary,
without whose love, help, patience, and support
this book would not have been written.

Published by Contemporary Books, Inc.
180 North Michigan Avenue, Chicago, Illinois 60601
Manufactured in the United States of America
Library of Congress Catalog Card Number: 87-19916
International Standard Book Number: 0-8092-4677-5

Published simultaneously in Canada by Beaverbooks, Ltd.
195 Allstate Parkway, Valleywood Business Park
Markham, Ontario L3R 4T8 Canada

# CONTENTS

# ACKNOWLEDGMENTS

The author is grateful to the writers and publishers listed below for permission to use and/or draw upon or adapt material from their publications in compiling and/or reproducing graphs and tables for use in this book:

*Figure 1, page 2.* Soules, MR, and Bremmer, WJ, "The Menopause and Climacteric: Endocrinologic Basis and Associated Symptomatology," *Journal of American Geriatrics Society,* 1982; 30:547-561. MTP Press Limited.

*Figure 2, p. 8.* Scott, JZ, "The Menopause," *Current Problems in Obstetrics, Gynecology and Fertility,* 1985; 8:1:21. Year Book Medical Publishers, Inc.

*Figure 5, p. 29, and Figure 7, p. 33.* Raisz, LG, "Clinical Recognition of Osteoporosis," *Osteoporosis: A Clinician's View,* May 1984, pp 3-4, Figures 2 and 3. Biomedical Information Corporation.

*Figure 8, p. 34.* Garroway, Wm, Stauffer, RN, Kurland, LT, and O'Fallon, WM, "Limb Fractures in a Defined Population. I. Frequency and Distribution," *Mayo Clinic Proceedings,* 1979; 54:701-707. Mayo Foundation.

*Figure 9, p. 36.* Christiansen, C, Christensen, MS, and Transbol, I, "Bone Mass in Postmenopausal Women After Withdrawal of Estrogen/Gestagen Replacement Therapy," *Lancet,* 1981; 1:459-461. Little, Brown & Co.

*Table 1, p. 45.* Ross, RK, et al, "Menopausal Oestrogen Therapy and Protection from Death from Ischaemic Heart Disease," *Lancet,* 1981; 1:858. Little, Brown & Co.

*Figure 10, p. 53, and Figure 11, p. 56.* Gambrell, RD, "Sex Steroid Hormones and Cancer," *Current Problems in Obstetrics and Gynecology,* October 1984; 114:27, 52. Year Book Medical Publishers, Inc.

*Figure 12, p. 71.* Buchsbaum, Herbert J, *The Menopause,* 1983; p. 2, Fig.1-1. Springer-Verlag.

*Figure 13, p. 84.* Hirvonen, E, Malkonen, M, Manninen, V, "Effects of Different Progestogens on Lipoproteins During Postmenopausal Replacement Therapy," *New England Journal of Medicine,* 1981; 304:560-563.

*Figure 3, p. 10, Figure 4, p. 28, and Figure 6, p. 32,* are the work of the author.

# INTRODUCTION

For centuries women have heard that the menopause is a natural occurrence. They have been taught to await the menopause with hopeful anticipation. When it arrives, they will no longer have to put up with the scourge, the monthly, the curse, the sickness: the menses. Women learn to look forward to the coming of the menopause.

Some physicians have been among those who have fostered the idea that menopause is normal and natural. When women have approached their physicians with various menopausal complaints such as hot flashes, depression, anxiety, and insomnia, some doctors have told them that these are the normal symptoms of menopause and will eventually pass. Or the doctors have given them various medications to temporarily "get them through" the menopause.

All these responses were not wrong. Physicians and family counseled women according to the accepted beliefs of the time. However, times have changed. Physically, mentally, and emotionally, the women of today are re-

1

Figure 1
Changes in Female Life Expectancy vs Age of Menopause

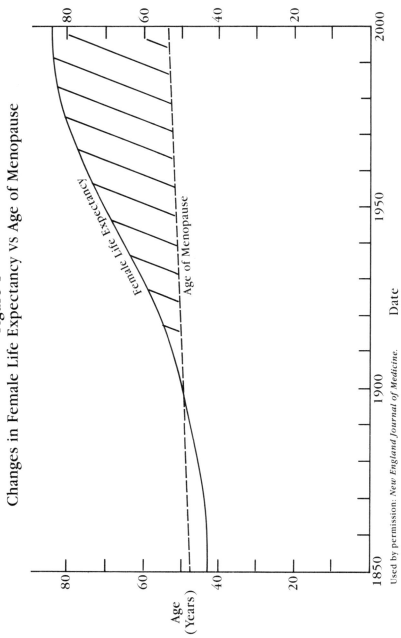

Female Life Expectancy

Age of Menopause

Age
(Years)

Date

markably different from those of yesterday. And if modern women want to take advantage of modern-day knowledge, they have to forget the old information about menopause.

Women of today are living much longer than ever before. It may be hard to believe that in 1900 the average life expectancy of a female living in the United States was only 48 years of age. This means that half of all women were dead by the age of 48. Today, as shown in Figure 1, a woman who has reached the age of 50 can, on the average, expect to live to the age of 85.

Although women are living much longer, the age of menopause has not changed proportionately. As shown in Figure 1, between the years 1900 and 1986, the average age of menopause has changed from 47 years to 51.4 years. This is an increase of only 4.4 years, compared to a 32-year increase in life expectancy. Women now live one-quarter to one-half of their lives after menopause. This fact makes women of today physically different from their female ancestors. It also suggests that menopause must be handled differently than it was in the past.

Today's woman also is significantly different mentally. Women are far better educated than ever before. This is especially true as far as their health is concerned. We are more aware of diseases, their treatments, and their prevention. We are aware of the dangers of excess weight, the advantages of regular exercise, and the importance of preventing disease or detecting it as early as possible. Today, women look for and use new medical findings to aid them in maintaining their health, nutrition, and appearance. This new knowledge gives modern women a mental edge over women of the past.

There has been a great emotional change in women. Modern women are more self-assured and self-reliant. Women today should not be, and usually are not, willing to accept menopause as a time of getting old, slowing down, or leaving the mainstream of life's activities. More women than ever are employed outside the home. They play much more aggressive roles in business and in their family lives. In many cases, their feelings about continuing an active sexual life during and after the menopause are much more liberal than those of past generations.

Women generally are unwilling to accept anxiety, depression, or lethargy as conditions they have to tolerate as they pass through the years surrounding the menopause. They are aware that chemical (hormonal) changes in their own bodies can radically affect their emotions. These chemical changes of the menopause can and do significantly change a woman emotionally. However, women are learning that available drugs will restore their chemical balance and thereby restore their emotional stability.

The following chapters present a series of questions about the menopause. You can peruse the book from beginning to end and get a complete picture of menopause, its symptoms, effects, and treatment. Or you can refer to the questions you want specific information about.

# 1
# MENOPAUSE
# AND LIFE STAGES

### *What is the menopause?*

The menopause is a point in time, not a duration of time. The menopause is that point in a woman's life after which she has no further menstrual flows (periods or menses). Physicians usually state that a woman is truly menopausal when she has gone without a menstrual flow for twelve months. (Some physicians use six months without flow.)

We cannot predict the actual age of menopause for a particular woman. Daughters tend to follow age trends similar to those of their mothers. This is especially true for those who tend to reach the menopause before the age of 40. No relationship has been shown between the age at which periods begin and the age of menopause.

Most physicians consider the average age of menopause for present-day women to be 50 years. As mentioned in the Introduction, the average age of menopause has slowly risen over the last 100 years from 47 years to 51.4 years. (At least 10 percent of all women will have already reached the menopause by the age of 40.) The probable reasons for this slow increase in the age of menopause include better nutrition, better living conditions, planned parenthood, and generally better health.

### What is the premenopause?

The premenopause is that period of life before the menopause (cessation of all menses). More commonly, when we refer to the premenopause, we are speaking about the years before the last menses when signs of menstrual irregularity and/or hot flashes are beginning. This usually represents the years between 40 and the menopause.

### What is the postmenopause?

The postmenopause is all the years of life remaining after the point of menopause (cessation of all menses). When most people refer to "the menopause," they are really speaking about the postmenopause. Most of the significant degenerative changes that are discussed in this book occur during this period of a woman's life and are directly related to the estrogen deficiency a woman develops due to failing ovaries. This is the time of life women have been taught to accept, but in reality they should be actively correcting their hormone deficiency.

### What is the perimenopause?

The perimenopause is the time immediately before and after the menopause. Usually this begins with the 12-month period before the menopause, when symptoms of change in hormonal balance begin, and ends 12 months after the menopause. When a woman speaks of the symptoms of "the menopause," she usually is referring to the symptoms that occur in the perimenopause. Remember, the menopause is a *point* in time, while the perimenopause is a *span* of time.

### What is the "change of life"?

As described earlier, the menopause is a dramatic point in time when a woman stops having all further cyclic menstrual flow. Most women go through a span of time during which they notice various changes. This span of time is often referred to as the "change of life." It varies in length from months to years before the menopause and from months to years after the menopause. Most women experience these changes, which result from fluctuating and decreasing hormone levels before and after the actual menopause. However, some women have none of these symptoms until after the periods stop, and a few have no symptoms at all.

This span of time is also referred to as "the climacteric years"—meaning the time that begins when the first signs of the approaching menopause occur and ends when the woman's last period occurs and her subjective symptoms eventually subside.

The general public most often refers incorrectly to this period as "the menopause." The correct term to use for this commonly discussed and often distressful period of life is the *perimenopause*.

In summary, "change of life," "the climacteric years," and "the perimenopause" are all used to describe the period of a woman's life when she experiences symptoms of hormonal deficiencies before and after the time of her last menses.

### Why does the menopause occur?

When a girl is born, she already has all the egg cells she will ever have in her ovaries: approximately 700,000 eggs. (This is remarkably different from the male, who has no sperm at birth. The manufacturing of sperm begins at puberty and continues until late in life, 70-80 years of age.) Females lose eggs between birth and puberty, so that at puberty the female has approximately

Figure 2

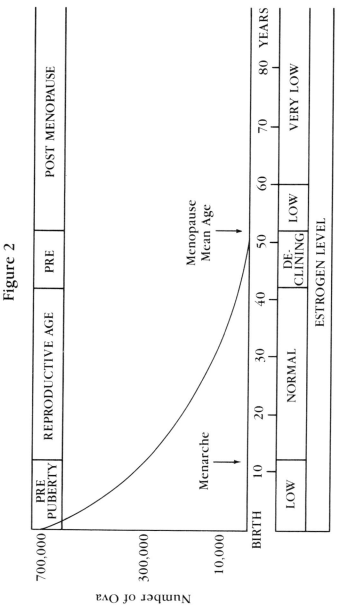

half (300,000-400,000) of the eggs with which she was born.

Estrogen is a hormone (chemical) that produces the major female characteristics. It is also vital to the development and maintenance of many tissues in the body. The breasts, bones, skin, bladder, and vagina are just a few of the structures that depend on estrogen. This hormone is manufactured mainly in the ovaries and, more specifically, the egg cells.

At the time of puberty, a series of chemical changes takes place in the female, causing her to begin regular cyclic maturation of eggs in the ovaries. This is more fully described under the next question, "What is the menstrual cycle?" The activation of the eggs and their maturation cycle (menstrual cycle) leads to increased levels of estrogen and, as a result, development of sexual characteristics.

With the onset of each menstrual cycle, many eggs begin to develop in each ovary. Usually they all die except one, which is extruded by the ovary at the time of ovulation. In this way, many eggs (20-1000) are used up each month. Eventually the ovary, for all practical purposes, becomes empty of eggs. At that time the ovary's estrogen production reaches such a low level that menstrual cycles and flow cease. The woman has reached menopause. See Figure 2 for an illustration of this description.

### What is the menstrual cycle?

As mentioned, the menstrual cycle usually begins at puberty. The time of puberty varies from female to female, but in general normal occurrence is considered to be between the ages of 10 and 18 years. The time of onset of menstrual cycles (menarche) is not significantly related to the time of onset of the menopause.

Figure 3
The Menstrual Cycle

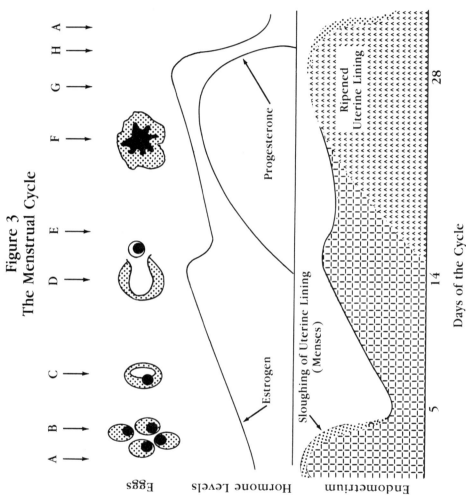

Figure 3 illustrates the stages of the menstrual cycle. The horizontal axis represents the days of the cycle. Medically speaking, the first day of the cycle refers to the first day of menstrual bleeding. It does not matter whether the flow is bright or dark, heavy or light, only that there has been a show of blood. At this time, the woman's estrogen level is very low. The lining of the uterus, which grew during the preceding cycle, is dying and shedding from the uterine walls. (See *A* in Figure 3.)

The normal menstrual flow lasts three to seven days. During these first few days of the cycle, many eggs in each ovary start to mature. (See *B* in Figure 3.) Their growth causes them to produce more and more estrogen. This increasing estrogen level (shown by the upper curve labeled Estrogen) causes the lining of the uterus to grow. The growth of the uterine lining is also represented day by day on the bottom curve of Figure 3.

By day 5-7 of the cycle, most of the eggs that began developing on the first day of the cycle are degenerating or have stopped developing. At this time, the strongest egg is developing rapidly and producing larger and larger amounts of estrogen (see *C*, Figure 3). On approximately the 14th day of the cycle, the egg cyst (follicle cyst) has reached maturity, and the egg within the cyst is expelled from the ovary; in other words, ovulation occurs (see *D*, Figure 3). The egg begins its journey into the fallopian tube and eventually reaches the uterus.

Interestingly, when the egg cyst ruptures and expels the egg, the function of the egg cyst may be disrupted enough to diminish the production of estrogen for a short time (approximately 24 hours). In some women, this drop in estrogen production can cause the lining of the uterus (the endometrium) to break down and bleed because it critically depends on estrogen for its growth and survival. This short-lived breakdown and bleeding is the cause of so-called midcycle (ovulatory) spotting (see *E*, Figure 3).

The egg cyst in which the egg developed collapses after the egg is expelled, and it develops into a new structure called a corpus luteum (see *F,* Figure 3). This new structure continues producing estrogen and also begins producing a second important female hormone called progesterone. This hormone could be called the "hormone of ovulation," since it is not produced in significant amounts unless ovulation has occurred. The production of progesterone increases rapidly, as shown in Figure 3 by the curve labeled Progesterone. The increasing levels of progesterone after ovulation cause the lining of the uterus to become "ripened" (see *G,* Figure 3).

If the egg formed and expelled during the cycle encounters sperm in the fallopian tube and becomes fertilized, a message (probably a chemical message) is sent to the corpus luteum, telling it that fertilization has occurred. If it receives this message, the corpus luteum continues to function, producing increasing levels of estrogen and progesterone in order to keep the lining of the uterus ripened for the implantation of a fertilized egg. The production of these high levels of estrogen and progesterone by the corpus luteum continues for the first 12-16 weeks of pregnancy, thereby maintaining the pregnancy until it is large enough to produce adequate levels of these hormones by itself.

If the egg formed and expelled during the cycle does not become fertilized, as in most cycles, a message (again, probably a chemical message) is sent to the corpus luteum, telling it that fertilization has not occurred. In this situation, the corpus luteum begins to degenerate, and the levels of estrogen and progesterone produced by the corpus luteum rapidly decrease (see *H,* Figure 3). With this decrease in the levels of estrogen and progesterone, the ripened lining dies and is shed from the walls of the uterus. This is the menses or period (see *A,* Figure 3). This "progesterone ripening" allows the uterus to empty rapidly and efficiently without excessive or prolonged uterine bleeding.

This description shows that ovulation followed by formation of a corpus luteum, which is followed by production of progesterone, is imperative for the development of a ripened uterine lining leading to a normal period. Without these occurrences, a woman's period is irregular.

# 2
# SIGNS OF MENOPAUSE

***What are the symptoms of the menopause?***

This question can be answered in several ways. There are those early symptoms or complaints which women are aware of and which are bothersome to them. There are also a number of significant effects on the female body that sometimes are not immediately apparent to the woman experiencing them.

The following list gives the most common complaints and the frequency with which they occur:

| *Complaint* | *%* |
|---|---|
| Irritability | 92 |
| Lethargy/fatigue | 88 |
| Depression | 78 |
| Headaches | 71 |
| Hot flashes | 68 |
| Forgetfulness | 64 |
| Weight gain | 61 |
| Insomnia | 51 |

| | |
|---|---|
| Joint pain/backache | 48 |
| Palpitations | 44 |
| Crying spells | 42 |
| Constipation | 37 |
| Burning upon urination | 20 |
| Decreased sex drive | 20 |

Many of these complaints will be discussed more fully under other questions.

The effects that are not immediately apparent (the silent changes) are actually more significant and medically important to the woman than are the early symptoms just listed. Some of the silent changes that start with the onset of the menopause are loss of calcium from the bones (osteoporosis), increased rate of hardening (narrowing) of the arteries (arteriosclerosis), thinning of the vaginal and bladder lining (atrophy), and the increased risk of uterine and breast cancer.

These symptoms and effects are discussed further on the following pages.

### What are the most common early signs of the menopause?

In most cases, the earliest signs of the approaching menopause are changes in the menstrual pattern. Not all changes in the menstrual pattern signify the approach of the menopause. There are many causes for irregular menses in prepubertal girls, girls at the time of puberty, women during the child-bearing years, and even postmenopausal women. However, changes in the menstrual pattern in a woman who is approaching the average age of menopause are most commonly the first signs of the approaching menopause.

These changes in the menstrual pattern may vary. The interval between periods may increase, or it may decrease. Changes can also take the form of heavier periods, lighter periods, shorter periods, longer periods, and occasionally spotting between periods. *Spotting between periods is a significant symptom in all women and should always be brought to the attention of a physician.*

The answers to two questions, "Why does the menopause occur?" and "What is the menstrual cycle?" will help you understand the following explanation of the causes of menstrual irregularity.

Around the age of 40, egg maturation begins to occur less frequently. At this time, probably only a few thousand eggs remain in the ovaries. This is a remarkable decrease from the approximately 400,000 eggs in the ovaries at the time of puberty. Because of this small number of eggs remaining in the ovaries, ovulation is often irregular.

All of the maturing eggs in a cycle may die, leading to an early decrease in estrogen production. The uterine lining (endometrium) depends on estrogen for its growth and survival. When the estrogen level drops significantly, the uterine lining dies and menstrual flow occurs. Because this lining was not ready to come out (was unripened), the flow may be abnormal (short, long, heavy, or light), as well as early.

At other times, no single maturing egg becomes dominant, and ovulation does not occur. In this case, estrogen is produced at an adequate level to sustain the uterine lining. In fact, because estrogen continues to be produced without ovulation and subsequent formation of progesterone, the lining of the uterus may be stimulated for much longer periods than normal and may become unusually thick (hyperplastic). When estrogen production finally stops for that cycle, the long-overdue menses will probably be heavy and prolonged. Clots commonly occur with this type of period.

At still other times, the start of the cycle or the time of ovulation may be delayed. In these cases, when ovulation does occur, the remainder of the cycle is usually normal. With ovulation, progesterone formed by the postovulation cyst (corpus luteum) ripens the uterine lining. Although the period may be long overdue, it is often normal in amount and duration.

Eventually, the few eggs remaining in the ovaries cannot be stimulated to mature. At this point, estrogen is produced at such a low level that it is insufficient to stimulate growth of the uterine lining. This is the point of menopause, the end of cyclic uterine bleeding.

### What is a hot flash?

The terms *hot flash*, *hot flush*, and *night sweat* all refer to the same phenomenon. Most women describe a hot flash as the sudden onset of a warm feeling in the face, neck, and chest. The hands also can be affected, but to a lesser degree than the other areas. The face develops a red flush, and the face, neck, and chest perspire. These episodes can last from seconds to several minutes. Some women find them exceedingly uncomfortable, and at times the flashes may be accompanied by nausea, headaches, or dizziness. They initially seem to occur more often in the evenings and at night. However, as women progress further into the early postmenopausal period, the hot flashes become more severe, longer, more frequent, and can occur at any time of the day or night.

About 85 percent of women experience hot flashes in the perimenopausal period. The majority (75 percent) of women continue to experience these uncomfortable episodes for more than a year. Fewer than 25 percent of women suffer with them beyond five years.

This period of menopausal symptoms can be likened to the period of withdrawal seen in addicts. Basically, the body is experiencing withdrawal from estrogen, just as an addict experiences withdrawal from a narcotic. The tissues of the body interact with estrogen from the time of puberty, and they develop a certain dependency on estrogen. When the estrogen level falls to a certain critical, low level, the body tissues react to the lack of estrogen, and the hot flashes begin.

The physiological cause of these hot flashes is not yet determined. However, we do know that the lack of estrogen causes an instability in the body mechanism that controls the blood vessels. This instability in control opens blood channels suddenly, causing a surge of blood to the surface of the skin in the areas of the face, neck, chest, and hands. This leads to the warm feeling, flushing, and sweating in those areas.

### What about "emotional changes" during the perimenopause?

Depression, anxiety, crying spells, and irritability are all emotional changes that occur in the perimenopause (climacteric years). All too often, women are told that these symptoms are "attitude," "all in your head," "just your imagination," or "just your nerves acting up." For years physicians believed that if a woman had a well-balanced life and had properly prepared herself for her later years, she would not experience any of these emotional symptoms in the postmenopausal years.

Many excellent studies now indicate that low levels of estrogen occurring in the perimenopausal years *do* have a definite physiological effect on important centers in the brain. In addition to hot flashes, the "withdrawal" from estrogen causes changes in the brain, which affect a woman's thought processes and lead to depression, anxiety, irritability, forgetfulness, insomnia, crying spells, lethargy, and fatigue. These are not the symptoms of the woman who is ill-prepared for the menopause or the symptoms of a psychologically weak person. They are hormonally caused and have a physiological basis.

Like hot flashes, these symptoms decrease in intensity the further the woman progresses into the menopause. Her body adapts to the decrease in estrogen, and she survives the "withdrawal phase." However, if a woman does nothing to correct her estrogen deficiency, she will remain at a new lower level of emotional and physical functioning. She may adjust to this new low level of functioning and even accept it as the norm, but she will be worse off than if the deficiency were corrected.

This is not to say that women who are emotionally stable and who have developed multiple areas of interest do not fare well in these troublesome early years of the postmenopause. Indeed, they are able to adapt more readily and with milder emotional symptoms than women without many areas of interest. But even well-prepared women end up living at a lower level of emotional and physical functioning if they do not correct their estrogen deficiency.

### Can women become pregnant around the age of menopause?

The answer to the question "Why does the menopause occur?" (Chapter 1) stated that the number of eggs in a woman's ovaries decreases significantly as she approaches the point of menopause. As the total number of eggs decreases, the likelihood of ovulation decreases. When ovulation does not occur, pregnancy is impossible. However, in some women the irregularity in ovulation may go on for months or even years. Therefore, a woman at the age of menopause may go through a year or more without having a period, yet she may occasionally ovulate without warning.

If sperm have been deposited in the vagina within 48 hours of ovulation, pregnancy is possible. Thus, a woman who has not menstruated in six months or more may erroneously believe she has passed through the menopause and is therefore safe from pregnancy. This may not be true.

In conclusion, the woman who has gone at least 12 months without a period or who is older than the average age of menopause (51.4 years) and has not had a period for six months or longer has an extremely small chance of becoming pregnant, but it is not an impossibility.

# 3
# THE SILENT CHANGES

*What are the silent changes of the postmeno-pause?*

For all practical purposes, the symptoms that have already been discussed concerning the approaching menopause or, more correctly, the perimenopause, have been changes that occur just before or immediately after the menopause. These are particularly obvious and irritating to the woman experiencing them. However, other changes occur far more slowly and less obviously. These changes are:

- Atrophy
- Osteoporosis
- Arteriosclerosis
- Endometrial (uterine) cancer
- Breast cancer

Many tissues in the female body are sensitive to, and dependent on, the "female hormone" estrogen. In addition to the tissues involved in reproduction (such as the breasts, uterus, ovaries, and vagina), even the more basic tissues, such as bones, blood vessels, skin, and bladder are significantly affected by low levels of estrogen.

Although such symptoms as menstrual irregularities, absence of menstruation, hot flashes, anxiety, depression, and insomnia are more noticeable and irritating to the woman in the perimenopausal period, they are really not the important changes as far as the woman's future health and life are concerned.

As described earlier, these early symptoms are the effects of estrogen deficiency. They will in time spontaneously disappear as the woman's body adapts to the lack of estrogen. This cessation of the early symptoms of menopause is what a woman is talking about when she states, "I am through the change of life," or, "I got through the bad part of the menopause." Many women are falsely reassured by the disappearance of symptoms. At this time, they frequently stop seeking help for the menopause.

Women are led into a false sense of security, thinking that the disappearance of symptoms indicates they have made it through "the change" and are safe. In reality, the opposite is true. Although the perimenopausal symptoms they experienced were indeed uncomfortable and often difficult to cope with, they did not have serious consequences for the women's health. The later, slow-to-appear, so-called "silent effects" of the menopause have serious consequences on the health of the untreated postmenopausal woman. Because these later, silent effects of the menopause develop slowly and insidiously, women do not associate their changes with the estrogen deficiency of the postmenopause. They often blame the aging process for the changes in their vagina, bladder, skin, and supportive tissues, as well as unexpected fractures, increased rate of heart attacks, breast cancer, and uterine cancer. In reality, a good portion of these changes is caused or aggravated by an estrogen deficiency.

The following questions discuss the silent changes that occur in the postmenopause.

## What is atrophy?

According to the medical dictionary, atrophy is an acquired reduction in the size of a cell, tissue, organ, or region of the body. The types of atrophy relevant to a discussion of the menopause are atrophic changes in the vagina, bladder, and skin. Atrophy basically is a thinning and weakening of these tissues.

## What is atrophic vaginitis?

The mucous membrane lining of the vagina is sensitive to estrogen. In fact, the strength or thickness of the vaginal lining is directly related to the woman's estrogen level. The estrogen-sensitive area also includes the area of skin around the opening of the vagina (introitus). Because of the relatively low levels of estrogen in children before puberty, these vaginal areas are very thin. When a child is examined, the tissue around the opening of the vagina thus looks red and irritated. This thin, weaker lining in children allows the area to become irritated easily, causing the child to rub or scratch the genital area. It is also why children can easily develop an infection in this area, such as a yeast infection.

As a woman passes through puberty, she produces increasing levels of estrogen. This causes the vaginal lining and the area around the vaginal opening to thicken. Conversely, as the woman passes through the menopause and estrogen levels decline, the vaginal lining becomes thin and weak. These postmenopausal, degenerative changes in the mucous membrane of the vagina can lead to itching, irritation, discharge, and sometimes bleeding. This common disorder, found in postmenopausal women who are not on replacement hormones, is called atrophic vaginitis.

Atrophic vaginitis is common in postmenopausal women. Most often, the woman will complain to her physician that intercourse has become uncomfortable and irritating. She may have noticed some bleeding after intercourse. Other complaints may center around a burning sensation, itching, and sometimes a vaginal discharge. The vaginal lining in these women has become so thin that the mild trauma that occurs from the rubbing of the walls of the vagina during intercourse will cause an irritation. These symptoms may also occur even if the woman is not sexually active. If certain organisms are present, the vagina can become infected. This is one of the reasons that postmenopausal women are more susceptible to vaginal infections such as monilia (yeast), trichomonas, and bacteria.

Studies of the vaginal changes in the postmenopausal female have shown that not only do the cells making up the lining of the vagina change, but the blood circulation in the wall of the vagina also decreases. In addition, there is a measurable decrease in the quantity of vaginal secretions. These vaginal secretions, which are usually acidic in the young and healthy female, become neutral or even alkaline in the untreated postmenopausal woman. All of these changes lead to the irritating symptoms just discussed.

**Note:** Treatment of the condition of vaginal mucous membrane atrophy in the postmenopausal woman is very effective. Use of either oral estrogens or estrogen vaginal cream rapidly repairs the cells of the vaginal lining, restores the vaginal secretions, and makes them more acidic. It also increases the circulation to the vaginal lining.

### How does the menopause affect the bladder?

The mucous membrane lining of the bladder is also dependent on, and sensitive to, estrogen, although it is less sensitive than the vaginal lining. Changes in the bladder lining occur later in the menopause and require lower levels of estrogen than do the changes in the vagina.

When the mucous membrane lining of the bladder

degenerates as a result of low estrogen levels, the woman experiences frequent urination, urgency to urinate, and often burning or stinging with urination. The reasons for these symptoms are the same as discussed for the vagina. The thinner, weakened bladder lining is more susceptible to irritation and infection. Therefore, bladder infections are more common in postmenopausal women.

Treatment with oral estrogens reverses the atrophic changes of the bladder lining and relieves the urinary symptoms, as well as decreasing the frequency of bladder infections.

### What are the postmenopausal changes in the supportive tissues?

Connective tissue is one of the various types of tissue found in the human body. It includes such categories as cartilage, bones, and connective tissue proper. In general, it is considered supportive tissue. An important component of these supportive tissues is collagen. This substance makes up tough fibers that give support to surrounding cells because they resist stretching. Collagen is found in bone, skin, cartilage, and in loose and dense types of connective tissue proper.

Recent studies, as reported by Dr. Mark Brincat of King's College Hospital, London, have shown that low estrogen levels cause collagen concentration in supportive tissues to decrease. The decrease in collagen content weakens the basic supportive structure of the tissue, allowing it to sag. This shows up as wrinkling of the skin; sagging of the skin of the arms, legs, chin, and breasts; and sagging of the vagina, bladder, and rectum.

Studies have concluded that decreased estrogen leading to decreased collagen is a direct cause of thinning of the skin in postmenopausal women. Skin in an untreated woman is 50 percent thinner after she has been in the postmenopause six years. Further, estrogen replacement in the postmenopause increases the collagen content of the skin 36 percent. This slows the wrinkling, sagging, and thinning of the tissues.

The combination of loss of collagen content, stretching of vaginal and uterine supportive tissues during childbirth, thinning of the vaginal lining due to estrogen loss, and general degeneration of tissues through aging frequently lead to significant sagging of the vagina and/or uterus; this is called pelvic outlet relaxation. It can lead to protrusion (prolapse) of the bladder, rectum, or uterus through the vaginal opening. Prolapse of the bladder can lead to loss of urine with straining by jumping, running, coughing, or sneezing. Prolapse of the rectum can cause difficulty with having a bowel movement.

Postmenopausal women who receive estrogen replacement therapy show fewer signs of wrinkling of the skin and sagging of the skin on the neck, arms, breasts, and thighs. They also have less trouble with loss of support of the vagina, bladder, and rectum than women who are not on hormonal replacement therapy.

### What is osteoporosis?

Osteoporosis is the loss of calcium from bone. In general, there are three categories of osteoporosis: pathological, senile, and postmenopausal osteoporosis.

Pathological osteoporosis is related to a disease that interferes with the processes of bone production and bone absorption. This causes loss of calcium content of bone.

Senile osteoporosis can best be defined as age-related bone loss. It is well documented that this type of bone loss occurs in both men and women. It seems to result from an increase in the rate at which bone tissue breaks down (resorbs) that is not met by an equal increase in bone formation. More than likely, the major cause of senile osteoporosis is impaired formation of bone cells as a result of aging.

In contrast, postmenopausal osteoporosis is character-ized by a remarkable increase in bone loss after the menopause. This loss is directly related to increased bone resorption rather than to slower bone formation. One out of three postmenopausal women are afflicted by osteoporosis.

### What are the specific causes of osteoporosis in the postmenopause?

Calcium deficiency and reduced estrogen levels play a significant role in causing postmenopausal osteoporosis. Present-day studies indicate that in this type of osteopo-rosis, the major cause is an increase in the rate at which bone tissue breaks down (resorbs).

Reduced estrogen levels in postmenopausal women are associated with accelerated bone loss in the long bones of their arms and legs, as well as in the bones of their spine and pelvis. Although decreased estrogen levels are definitely related to increased bone resorption, we do not know exactly why decreased estrogen has this effect. The mechanism of estrogen control may be calcitonin regulation.

Calcitonin is a hormone common to men and women. It is known as a calcium-regulating hormone. Calcitonin directly opposes bone resorption. Reduced levels of estrogen cause the secretion of calcitonin to decrease, which in turn accelerates the pace of bone resorption. Regulation of calcitonin secretion is thought to be the main mechanism by which estrogen protects women's bones.

Several additional factors probably have a direct effect on the more rapid bone loss in postmenopausal women. Calcium intake in the U.S. population is, in general, low. The average dietary intake of calcium in females over the age of 35 in the United States is 0.5 gram per day. Medical studies have shown that the average postmenopausal female not on estrogen replacement therapy loses 1.5

grams of calcium a day. Thus, women in the United States need to supplement their diet with at least 1 gram of calcium a day (see Figure 4). For additional information concerning calcium, see the questions "How can post-menopausal osteoporosis be prevented or treated?" and "Are there differences among calcium supplements?" later in this chapter.

Calcium replacement is not the entire answer for treatment of postmenopausal osteoporosis. Even among

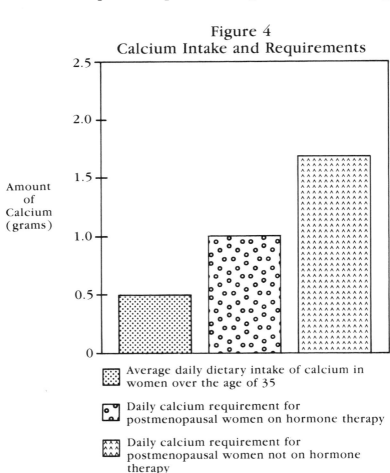

Figure 4
Calcium Intake and Requirements

Amount of Calcium (grams)

▦ Average daily dietary intake of calcium in women over the age of 35

◖◙◗ Daily calcium requirement for postmenopausal women on hormone therapy

▨ Daily calcium requirement for postmenopausal women not on hormone therapy

women taking adequate calcium, those not on replacement estrogen lose more bone tissue than those taking estrogen replacements.

The level of vitamin D also seems to decrease in the postmenopausal woman. This may lead to a decrease in intestinal absorption of calcium.

Collagen is an important component of bones and is directly related to their strength. As in skin, the collagen content of bone decreases in direct relationship to the decrease in estrogen level during postmenopause. The loss of collagen from bones is correctable with estrogen replacement.

Men have a greater bone mass than women, because similar bones are bigger and thicker in men than in women. Further, many studies have shown that the rate of bone formation is similar in men and women until the age of menopause (see Figure 5). At that time, women's bones begin to resorb much faster.

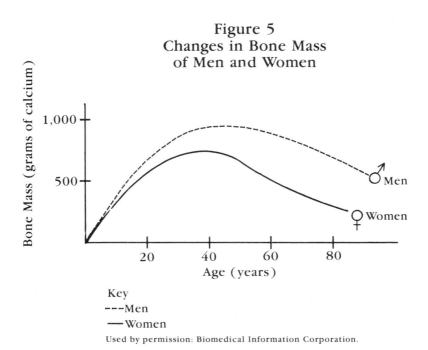

Figure 5
Changes in Bone Mass
of Men and Women

Key
---Men
—Women

Used by permission: Biomedical Information Corporation.

The curves in Figure 5 show the difference in the rates at which bone mass decreases between the ages of 40 and 70, with women losing bone mass much more rapidly than men. After the age of 70, the rates of bone loss again become parallel, but the difference in total bone mass between men and women has increased. Thus, men end up with a proportionately larger bone mass.

The difference in bone resorption between men and women leads to a remarkable increase in bone problems in women. Testosterone in men, like estrogen in women, seems to slow down bone resorption. While men experience no remarkable decrease in the male sex hormone until late in life, women's loss of estrogen leads quickly and directly to loss of calcium from bone. Therefore, resorption of bone is much less in older men than in older (postmenopausal) women.

### What problems does osteoporosis cause in the menopause?

As already mentioned, osteoporosis in its simplest definition is loss of bone tissue. Bones are made up of protein fibers (collagen) combined with calcium salt crystals. This combination gives bones their strength. Loss of bone protein and calcium weakens bones. In long bones, the marrow spaces (center cavities) get larger, while the cortex (outer shell) of bone thins.

Osteoporosis takes its toll in the form of fractures and impairment of skeleton functions. The disease is usually undetected until a fracture occurs. Most commonly, the fracture is unexpected. This type of fracture is termed a "pathological fracture," meaning that it occurred because of an underlying defect in the bone.

Osteoporosis is a common and serious disease and is a major health problem among menopausal women. It often goes undetected until it is in advanced stages. No simple or inexpensive tests exist to detect it early in its course. Surprisingly, it is a major cause of death in postmenopausal women. Although women probably worry more about cancer of the uterus than about fractures, 150 times more deaths result from fractures in menopausal women than from cancer of the uterus.

Osteoporosis problems fall into two major categories: one involving the long bones, and the other the vertebrae. Each type will be discussed separately.

The vertebral column is like a stack of building blocks that support the skeleton. It allows you to stand erect in a straight line. As the mineral and protein content of the vertebrae decreases, and subsequently their strength, compression fractures can occur in the main bodies of the vertebrae (see Figure 6).

These fractures begin early in the postmenopausal years and grow more frequent with age. The damage is seldom identifiable. It is estimated that 25 percent of women over the age of 60 who are not on hormonal replacement will have one or more vertebral fractures. Progressive loss of height and increasing deformity occur as more and more vertebrae are compressed.

This is demonstrated in Figure 7. The skeleton in *A* represents that of a young woman during the reproductive years. *B* represents the shortening skeleton of a woman after the first 10 years of menopause. *C* represents a woman in her 70s or beyond. The women represented in this figure have not had estrogen replacement. Note the increasing number of collapsed vertebrae in the aging female and the increasing prominence of the "dowager's hump." An untreated, postmenopausal, white female can expect to lose an average of 1.5 inches in height. As shown in Figure 7, the overall loss in height may amount to as much as 3.5 inches as a result of these compression fractures of the vertebrae.

Other problems caused by osteoporosis are outward curving of the upper back and protuberance of the abdomen. Not only are these changes disfiguring, they

# Figure 6
## Compression Fractures of
## Vertebrae of the Neck

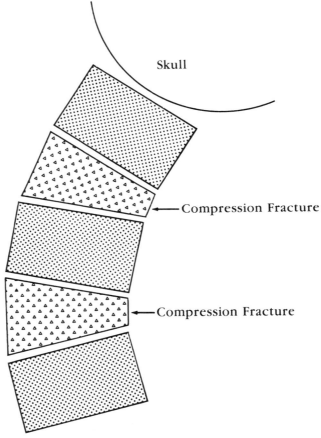

**Note:** The rectangles represent the main bodies of the
vertebrae of the neck. The deformed rectangles
(trapezoids) represent vertebrae that have sustained
compression fractures, thereby causing the upper vertebrae to
be curved.

## Figure 7
## Vertebral Crush Fracture Syndrome

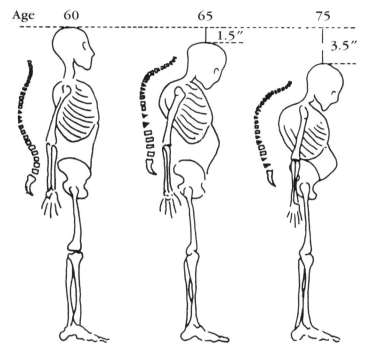

Used by permission: Biomedical Information Corporation.

Progressive loss of height and increasing deformity occur as more and more vertebral bodies are compressed.

can cause pain. In severe cases, women may complain of abdominal discomfort and pain resulting from the pressure of the ribs on the pelvic bone.

Common problems related to these spinal compression fractures include dysfunction of the lungs, bladder, stomach, and digestive system. Acute pain may occur and last for several weeks after a vertebral crush fracture. Chronic back pain can also occur. In some cases, this develops slowly without an identifiable acute episode. These symptoms are five times more common in women than men.

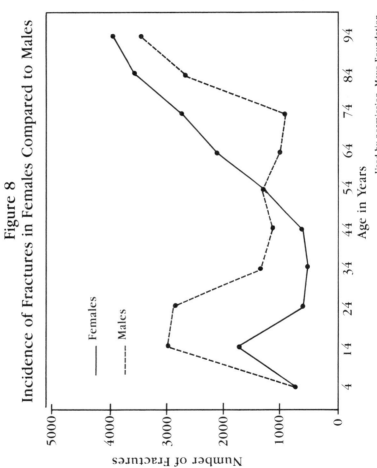

Figure 8
Incidence of Fractures in Females Compared to Males

Fractures of the long bones occur later in life than vertebral fractures. The most common of these are hip fractures and fractures of the forearm. Figure 8 shows the rates of bone fracture in men and women according to age. As expected, the rates of fracture in men and women increase through the teenage years and peak in the 20s. Also as expected, fractures occur more frequently among men than among women. These findings reflect the aggressive physical activities (sports and physical labor) in these age groups, especially among men, who expose themselves to more risk of an accident.

As men and women enter their 30s, their fracture rate drops significantly. However, whereas men continue to have a low rate of bone fractures until they get into their late 70s, the women show a remarkable increase in their fracture rate in their late 40s. Furthermore, their fracture rate continues to increase into the postmenopausal years. The rate of fractures for men never again exceeds that of women. The difference is directly related to women's loss of bone strength caused by loss of calcium and bone protein. This, in turn, is related to decreased estrogen levels in postmenopausal women.

Figure 8 shows that women of 40 have a rate of 800 fractures per 100,000 population. By the age of 70, women have a rate of nearly 4,000 fractures per 100,000 population. In contrast, for men at the age of 70, the fracture rate is only 1,200 per 100,000 population. Looking at this another way, women in their 50s have less than a 5 percent chance of a long-bone fracture due to osteoporosis. In their 60s, women have approximately a 25 percent chance of such a fracture. In their 70s, women have a 50 percent chance of a fracture related to osteoporosis.

Many people think fractures are not a mortal danger. But hip fractures in postmenopausal women carry a high risk of death. Between 15 and 20 percent of patients with hip fractures die within three months because of the fracture or surgical, cardiopulmonary (heart or lung

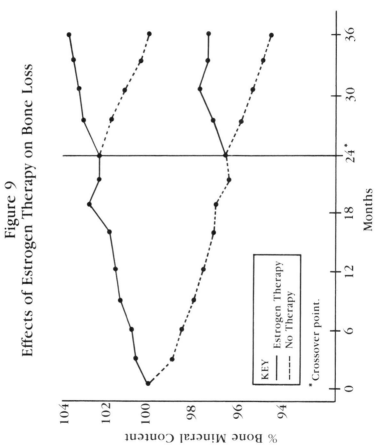

Figure 9
Effects of Estrogen Therapy on Bone Loss

Used by permission: Little, Brown & Co.

disease), or embolic (blood clots) complications. In addition, those who survive frequently are severely disabled the remainder of their life.

Certain factors predispose women to the development of osteoporosis:

- Early menopause (natural or surgical)
- Small, slender physique
- Family history of osteoporosis
- No children
- Race (Caucasian or Oriental)
- Smoking
- Abusive alcohol consumption
- Low calcium intake
- High caffeine intake
- High protein intake
- Inactive lifestyle
- Prolonged exposure to exogenous thyroid hormone
- Excessive exercise

Complete hysterectomy and early menopause are directly related to estrogen deficiency. So far we lack clear explanations for the remaining predisposing factors listed. Nevertheless, women should be aware of these factors and watch for signs of developing osteoporosis when they are present.

### How can postmenopausal osteoporosis be prevented or treated?

Commonly recommended medical treatments for postmenopausal osteoporosis include calcium supplements, vitamin D, fluoride, anabolic (tissue-building) agents, and exercise. However, no studies have shown that any of these treatments have as much effect on osteoporosis as does estrogen.

Figure 9 shows the results of a classic study of the corrective effect of estrogen therapy on bone loss in women who have had their ovaries removed. The vertical axis of the graph represents the percent of mineral content in bone. The lower curve represents the loss of mineral content of bone, and thereby the bone strength, in women who did not receive estrogen replacement therapy. When estrogen therapy is instituted in these women, the mineral content loss is stopped and in fact increases slightly.

The upper curve represents women who are immediately placed on estrogen replacement therapy when they enter their period of estrogen deficiency (after menopause or after surgery to remove both ovaries). The curve shows a maintenance or slight increase in bone mineral content. When estrogen replacement therapy is discontinued, the loss of mineral content of bones rapidly accelerates.

An important observation to make from this graph is that once a woman is allowed to lose the mineral content of bone because of lack of estrogen, estrogen replacement will not restore the mineral content to its level before the estrogen deficiency. This observation suggests that an aggressive approach to postmenopausal osteoporosis is necessary for two reasons. Therapy is more effective, the closer it is initiated to menopause. And once significant amounts of bone have been lost, complete retrieval can never be achieved.

The effect of estrogen replacement therapy on osteoporosis has been extensively studied over the past 30 years. Several definite, well-supported conclusions have resulted:

- Estrogen replacement therapy begun at the time of the menopause and continued for at least 10 years protects women from loss of central vertebral height. This includes protection from development of the so-called dowager's hump.
- The rate of fractures of the long bones (mainly hip and lower arm)—which increases from 5 percent in the 50s to 50 percent in the 70s—is decreased by 60 percent in all age groups when estrogen therapy has been carried out for six or more years.

• An estrogen dose equal to 0.625 milligram of Premarin (conjugated equine estrogens, see page 73) is necessary for the most efficient prevention of bone loss. Lower estrogen doses will be less effective. Higher estrogen doses do not increase efficiency, but they sometimes are necessary to adequately treat hot flashes and thinning of the linings of the vagina and the bladder.

Vitamin D supplements have been suggested as treatment for osteoporosis; however, research has not shown a significant effect on mineral content of bone or bone strength. In fact, therapeutic regimens of vitamin D have had the somewhat deleterious effect of excessive levels of calcium in the blood and urine. Women should consume adequate amounts of vitamin D, but excessive dosage may be counterproductive.

Sodium fluoride is a potent stimulator of bone formation. Combined with calcium and estrogen therapy, it increases the bone strength to the point of reducing osteoporotic fractures by 90 percent. However, there is a 40 percent rate of side effects with fluoride supplementation, including inflammation of joints and tendons, anemia, and disturbances of the stomach and digestive system. The recommended daily dose of sodium fluoride is 60 to 70 milligrams. The intake of calcium must be adequate, so that the new bone formed by stimulation of the fluoride will contain adequate minerals.

Contrary to old wives' tales, recent studies show that calcium requirements of the aging female are greater than previously realized. A national survey has shown that the average American woman over the age of 35 has a dietary calcium intake of 500 milligrams per day. With this consumption, the normal postmenopausal woman will lose 40 milligrams of calcium each day. The postmenopausal, estrogen-deficient woman requires 1.5 grams of calcium just to keep up with her daily loss. Women receiving estrogen replacement need only 1.0 gram of calcium per day to prevent loss of calcium. These facts indicate that neither estrogen alone nor calcium alone can prevent calcium loss.

Calcium supplementation along with estrogen replacement reduces the number of osteoporotic fractures by 80 percent in postmenopausal women. A combination of calcium, estrogen, and sodium fluoride will reduce the fracture rate by 90 percent. However, because of the side effects of fluoride supplementation, the most used regimen at present is a combination of calcium and estrogen.

Some recent studies presented at the 1984 Fourth International Congress on the Menopause described postmenopausal women who received cyclic progesterone along with estrogen and calcium. Contrary to expectations, not only did these women stop their bone loss, but they actually increased the mineral content of their bones. Previously, it was impossible to get increased mineral content in osteoporotic bone. The cyclic use of progesterone will be discussed later in the book.

Along with supplemental calcium, vitamin D, estrogen, and progesterone, exercise plays an important role in preventing osteoporosis. Women who participate in regular exercise programs show increased bone density and bone strength. Adequate exercise would include one of the following:

- Jogging 20 minutes 3-5 times a week
- Walking briskly 2-3 miles a day
- Bicycle riding 5-10 miles a day
- Aerobics 3-5 times a week

**Note:** Excessive exercise can lead to a loss of calcium from the bones.

### Are there differences among calcium supplements?

As far as the quality of the calcium obtained, one calcium tablet is about as good as another. But there is a big difference in the cost and amount of calcium available for absorption in the various tablets. It will take 10 calcium gluconate tablets at a cost of approximately $0.47 to get half a gram of calcium. Ten tablets of calcium lactate cost

$0.24 and also provide half a gram of calcium. With calcium carbonate, only two tablets provide a half-gram of calcium and cost $0.14. OS-CAL, a product made from oyster shells, contains half a gram of calcium in one tablet and costs only $0.09 per tablet. To most people's surprise, the least expensive and one of the easiest ways to get a half-gram of calcium is to chew two Tums tablets at a cost of $0.06. The chemical form of calcium you take is not important, but rather that you take enough tablets to equal the amount of calcium supplement you require.

Recently a controversy has arisen concerning whether Tums or Rolaids is a better calcium supplement for the prevention of osteoporosis. This issue is based on the different formulations of these antacids. Tums tablets contain calcium carbonate, while the calcium in Rolaids is connected to aluminum hydroxide. The only thing I have found to favor use of Tums over Rolaids is a report showing that aluminum-coating antacids such as Rolaids can cause phosphorus depletion accompanied by extensive calcium loss.

Another issue is whether their neutralizing of stomach acid impairs the absorption of calcium. Calcium is absorbed in an acid environment by being changed into calcium chloride, but Tums and Rolaids neutralize the acid. However, several studies have indicated that even when a person ingests large quantities of calcium carbonate (the ingredient in Tums), the amount of calcium absorbed is not decreased. In persons with impaired production of stomach acid, absorption is even facilitated when the Tums are ingested during a meal. *Note:* In postmenopausal women it is suggested the calcium be taken during a meal, when absorption is better.

### Who should be treated with estrogen and calcium replacement therapy?

Postmenopausal osteoporosis produces symptoms in 4 million women in the United States. Blood studies are not available to diagnose postmenopausal osteoporosis. X-rays and isotope tests are available for detecting it but only after up to 40 percent of bone mineral content has been lost. New, more sensitive tests (such as dual photon absorptiometry) are becoming more available, but these still are positive only after significant amounts of mineral content have been lost. The lost minerals cannot be retrieved by any proven existing therapy.

Prevention of osteoporosis in the aging woman is a major public health problem. Because of the large number of women living one-third of their life span in the postmenopausal state, the majority will at some time experience osteoporosis. Early postmenopausal estrogen and calcium therapy will significantly reduce osteoporosis. In turn, this reduction of osteoporosis will improve quality of life, reduce mortality, and save money.

Because we can never completely replace the mineral content of bone lost to osteoporosis, estrogen and calcium therapy must begin before the process has reached clinical significance, and it should continue into the woman's 70s. Perhaps asking who to treat is the wrong question. Maybe we should ask who we should not treat. Most women with estrogen deficiency can and should be treated with estrogen and calcium.

### How does the menopause affect arteriosclerosis?

Basically, atherosclerosis and arteriosclerosis are a plugging up and a hardening of the arteries. These changes are especially detrimental to the arteries of the heart and brain. Sudden plugging of the arteries of the heart causes a heart attack. Similar plugging of the arteries of the brain leads to stroke.

It has long been known that men have a greater incidence of heart attack than women of the same age. At the age of 50, a man is 6 times more likely to die from a heart attack than a woman of the same age. This is particularly noteworthy considering that a woman who has been in the postmenopause for 10 years has lost this advantage against heart attacks.

The changes in a woman that lead to this remarkable increase in the risk of heart attack are, in part, related to the estrogen deficiency of the postmenopause. Estrogen lowers blood cholesterol and protects the blood vessels against atherosclerosis.

Many years ago a study was performed with a group of men who had heart attacks before the age of 40. The study split these men into two similar groups. One group was treated for heart attacks in the usual manner. The second group received the same accepted therapy as the first group but also received therapeutic doses of estrogen. The group treated with the additional estrogen showed a remarkable decrease in the number of heart attacks and a lower death rate than the men who did not receive the estrogen. The problem with this hormone therapy was that it caused the men to develop female sex characteristics such as breasts, fatty deposits on the hips, and voice changes. As you can imagine, this was not acceptable to the male patients.

Although the effects of estrogen on cardiovascular disease has been debated for many years, there is increasing evidence that it provides protection. How does estrogen affect atherosclerosis?

The blood contains groups of fats known as high- and low-density lipoproteins. The low-density proteins have a high content of cholesterol, which they readily deposit into plaques in the walls of the blood vessels. The low-density lipoproteins (LDL) are therefore atherogenic (plaque-forming). The high-density lipoproteins (HDL), in contrast, have a low content of cholesterol and tend to absorb cholesterol from cells. They transport it to the liver, where it is processed and excreted. Therefore, not only does HDL tend not to form plaques, but it even tends to absorb cholesterol from plaques and to make the plaques smaller. Increased levels of HDL and decreased levels of LDL reduce the tendency of atherosclerosis to occur.

Studies have shown that estrogen causes the LDL to stay low and the HDL to increase. The estrogen in women during their reproductive years protects their blood vessels from atherosclerosis. The male hormone testosterone does not have the same effect, resulting in men's increased risk of early atherosclerosis and heart attack. That is why the use of estrogen therapy in the men prone to heart attacks decreased their cardiovascular disease.

The protective effect of estrogen is lost when a woman becomes estrogen-deficient after the menopause. Estrogen replacement in postmenopausal women would be expected to protect them from atherosclerosis and cardiovascular disease. Table 1 demonstrates one study showing the protective effect of estrogen from heart attack.

Table 1 was taken from a study published in 1981 showing the risk of death from heart attack under various conditions. When a patient has had a stroke or has hypertension, the risk of dying from a heart attack is three times greater than if these conditions are not present. Angina and previous heart attack increase the risk to six to seven times. Also noteworthy is the fact that smoking one pack of cigarettes a day causes a three times greater risk of death from a heart attack than not smoking.

Table 1 also shows the factors that seem to protect against heart attack causing death. As shown, moderate use of alcohol decreases the risk of heart attack to one-third of the risk of a nondrinker. However, more importantly, estrogen replacement therapy causes a 60 percent decrease in risk of death from heart attack in women compared to those not using hormone replacement therapy. Estrogen therapy even significantly decreases the risk of death by heart attack in people who would normally have an increased risk due to smoking. Many other studies show the same protective effect of estrogen against death from heart attack.

TABLE 1
Factors that Influence Risk of Death from Heart Attack

| Factors | Risk Ratio |
| --- | --- |
| Increased Risk of Death: | |
| Stroke | 3.43 |
| Hypertension | 3.24 |
| Angina | 6.57 |
| Myocardial infarction | 7.33 |
| Smoking 1 pack cigarettes per day | 3.33 |
| Decreased Risk of Death: | |
| Moderate alcohol use | 0.38 |
| Estrogen therapy | 0.43 |
| Estrogens and smoking | |
| More than 1 pack per day | 0.80 |
| Less than 1 pack per day | 0.58 |

Used by permission: Little Brown & Co.

## But don't birth control pills aggravate heart disease?

The majority of birth control pills are made up of a combination of estrogen-like and progesterone-like chemicals. Medical studies show a significant increase in the risk of cardiovascular disease for women who smoke, are over 30, and use birth control pills. These studies also show significant increases in cardiovascular disease in women who do not smoke but are over 35 and take the Pill.

Hormonal therapy suggested for the postmenopausal women is made up of cyclic estrogen and progesterone somewhat similar to birth control pills. With this in mind, one might conclude that if cyclic birth control pills cause increased cardiovascular disease in women over the age of 35, then cyclic hormone replacement therapy (HRT) in the menopause could also cause this problem in postmenopausal women. However, what appears obvious on first glance is not true when the problem is studied in detail.

What is the difference between the Pill and HRT? Birth control pills have 12-20 times more estrogen than the average amount used in postmenopausal hormone replacement therapy. Furthermore, estrogen decreases cardiovascular disease by increasing the circulation of high-density lipoproteins. (See the previous question.) Something else in the Pill besides estrogen must therefore cause the problem with cardiovascular disease.

The difference is the large and prolonged doses of progesterone-like drugs, which are in each of the 21 pills a woman takes each month. Studies have shown that progesterone has the detrimental effect on women of decreasing the number of high-density lipoproteins. This counteracts the benefit of the estrogen.

In postmenopausal HRT, the progesterone is taken for only 10-13 days each month and is less potent than the progesterone found in oral contraceptives. This dosage resembles the way the body produces progesterone during normal menstrual cycles. Taken this way, it has less detrimental effect on the levels of HDL.

## How can women avoid cardiovascular hardening of the arteries?

In 1980, 350,000 women died from cardiovascular hardening of the arteries or atherogenic disease. (Death from breast cancer for the same period was only 35,000.) It is important to try to limit the risk of cardiovascular atherogenic disease. Although HRT is an important mechanism for protection against atherosclerosis in the menopause, several other practices will help prevent cardiovascular disease.

Change of lifestyle is an important way to decrease the risk of cardiovascular disease. Ways to protect your health when entering mid- and late-life include avoiding stressful business and personal situations, getting adequate rest, and avoiding severe physical stress.

Dietary habits are also important. A healthy diet limits cholesterol and fatty acids. Proper diet for weight control is also crucial. For each ten pounds you are over your ideal weight, you put your heart under a great deal of additional strain.

Smoking is an absolute killer. Smoking undeniably is directly linked to increased cardiovascular disease and death.

Finally, but far from least important, is a regular exercise program. Such an exercise program should include one of the following:

- Jogging 20 minutes 3-5 times a week
- Walking briskly 2-3 miles a day
- Bicycle riding 5-10 miles a day
- Aerobics 3-5 times a week

# 4
# HORMONES AND
# CANCER

## *What about hormones and uterine cancer?*

In the 1960s and 1970s, there was a great cancer scare concerning women taking hormones, especially estrogen. The Food and Drug Administration (FDA) began requiring pharmacists to hand out a sheet discussing the relationship of cancer to intake of estrogen (see Appendix A). This single act by the FDA has caused more damage to the female population in the USA than any other in the FDA's history. This cancer warning sheet frightened hundreds of thousands of women away from taking hormones. Even though we now have information to show the benefits of hormones in the menopause, the FDA has not seen fit to rewrite the warning sheet.

Because the FDA cancer statement is so negative about hormones, it has become a pet peeve of mine. The major portion of its statement relates to three independent studies reporting an increased risk of uterine (endometrial) cancer in postmenopausal women exposed to estrogen therapy for more than one year. The studies are valid. The problem with the statement is that it is limited only to a single bad side effect and does not tell of the advantages of estrogen therapy in postmenopausal women.

For instance, if the patient is going to be told that taking estrogens in the menopause for longer than a year is going to increase her risk of uterine cancer, she should also be told that if she denies herself estrogen therapy in the postmenopausal years, she runs a great risk of developing severe osteoporosis, which can lead to bone fractures, which cause 250 times more deaths in postmenopausal women than does uterine cancer. Patients should also be told that women who take estrogen in the postmenopause live on an average three to four years longer than women who do not take estrogens in the postmenopause. Although less convincing, there is also the fact that uterine cancers that develop in women who are on estrogen are found earlier, are more superficial, and have a higher cure rate than endometrial cancers that occur in women not taking estrogen.

The advantages of taking estrogen in the postmenopause are so much greater than the risk, that even if the estrogen is taken in the old-fashioned way, as it was in the studies presented by the FDA, the woman is better off taking estrogen than not. Most importantly, it is now known that the increased risk of uterine cancer can be reversed with the addition of cyclic progesterone therapy.

The FDA statement has not been kept up to date with these new findings on the treatment of the postmenopause and the use of estrogen-progesterone cycles, which actually decrease the risk of uterine cancer below that of women not taking estrogen. The studies on which the FDA based its statements were conducted many years ago when hormone replacement therapy was not well understood or tested. At that time, many physicians simply gave their patients a bottle of estrogen tablets and told them to take one a day, or one a day for 21 days each month. When postmenopausal women take estrogens in this fashion, they may overstimulate the growth of the uterine lining.

When the lining of the uterus is exposed to estrogen, it is stimulated to grow. Small doses of estrogen stimulate the lining to grow slowly; larger doses stimulate the lining to grow rapidly. If the lining is not cyclically exposed to progesterone to prepare it for a period, then the lining is not allowed to completely slough off the uterine wall during menses. When sloughing of the uterine lining does not occur or is incomplete, it builds up. Eventually the amount of estrogen being ingested by the woman is inadequate to support this thickened lining. At that point the woman begins to bleed irregularly or heavily. See the question "What is the menstrual cycle?" (Chapter 1).

Stimulation of the uterine lining for long periods of time (months or years) without exposure to cyclic progesterone and thereby cyclic emptying can overstimulate the cells making up the lining. This chronic overstimulation can lead to development of a cancer of the uterine lining in susceptible women. Approximately one-third of postmenopausal women receiving estrogen therapy without cyclic progesterone will develop overstimulation changes in the uterine lining. Of these severe cases of overstimulation, 10-30 percent will progress to a cancer within three or four years.

However, if the woman takes cyclic progesterone (5-10 milligrams a day for 10-13 days) at the end of each estrogen cycle, she will shed the lining at the end of each cycle and avoid the problems of uterine cancer and overstimulation changes. Adequate scientific studies conclusively show that not only will cyclic estrogen-progesterone treatment in postmenopausal women avoid increasing the risk of uterine cancer, but will actually protect women against it.

In the journal *Current Problems in Obstetrics and Gynecology*, R. Don Gambrell, Jr., M.D., summarizes what is probably the true relationship of replacement hormone therapy and endometrial cancer. Dr. Gambrell's study divided postmenopausal women into three basically similar groups. One group of women preferred to enter menopause and remain in the postmenopause without any hormone replacement therapy (HRT). The second group of women used estrogen-only therapy (no progesterone). The women in the third group were treated with cyclic estrogen and progesterone. As expected, this third group continued to have cyclic menses, thereby emptying the uterus each month. These three groups are depicted in Figure 10.

The group of women who received no hormone therapy had an endometrial cancer rate of 258 cases per 100,000 women. The group receiving estrogen-only therapy showed an incidence of 411 cancers per 100,000 women. This is almost double that of the group receiving no hormones. It is on this group that the FDA bases its warning concerning estrogen and endometrial cancer.

The third group received cyclic estrogen-progesterone therapy. This group showed more than a 50 percent *decrease* in the rate of endometrial cancer compared to the group taking no hormones. The rate of endometrial cancer was 68 cases per 100,000 women. This remarkable decrease in the rate of endometrial cancer is expected based on the knowledge that cyclic use of progesterone causes cyclic emptying of the uterus.

As described under the question, "What are the most common early signs of the menopause?" (Chapter 2), heavy or prolonged bleeding can result from continued estrogen production by the ovaries when there is absence of ovulation and thereby the absence of progesterone production. If for years after she stops ovulating, a woman continues to produce estrogen from various sources, including the failing ovaries, the liver, the skin, and the adrenal glands, the lining of her uterus may be slowly stimulated for months and years after the last

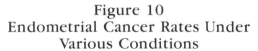

Figure 10
Endometrial Cancer Rates Under
Various Conditions

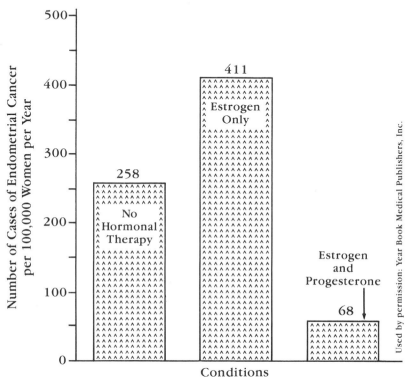

menses. This prolonged stimulation can, and often does, lead to an overstimulated uterine lining and eventually to uterine cancer. Since each woman has a different biochemistry, ancestry, diet, and level of activity, the amount of overstimulation varies, as does the tendency to develop uterine cancer.

Before leaving this subject of estrogen and increased risk of uterine cancer, let us look at the problem in a different way. Pretend that we did not know about or have progesterone to protect against development of uterine cancer. If we treated with estrogen alone, we would have to live with the FDA findings of a higher rate of uterine cancer. How could we rationalize using hormones in the face of this increased threat of cancer?

First, there is the fact that 250 times more women die in the menopause from bone fractures due to osteoporosis related to estrogen deficiency than die from uterine cancer. This means that a woman is better off taking the estrogens and risking the cancer than risking loss of calcium and osteoporosis and the high rate of death from fractures.

Second, studies that have compared women who did not take HRT to those who did found that no matter whether they took estrogen alone or estrogen-progesterone, those on HRT live an average of 3.5 years longer than those who did not take HRT.

And last, in women who did take estrogen alone and did develop an endometrial cancer, the cancer was usually found early, was usually superficial, and was unlikely to have spread. These characteristics lead to a cure rate of 80-90 percent. This is a higher cure rate than in uterine cancers that occur in women not on hormones.

The importance of treatment with estrogen alone in the postmenopausal woman who cannot take progesterone will be discussed in later questions.

This discussion is designed to dispel superstitions about hormones and uterine cancer. Don't miss further "good news" about hormones and breast cancer under the question "What about hormones and breast cancer?" later in this chapter.

### What about hormones and ovarian cancer?

There is no evidence that postmenopausal hormone replacement therapy (HRT) has any effect on the incidence of ovarian cancer. It is interesting to note that women who have taken birth control pills during the child-bearing years have a 40 percent reduction in ovarian cancer in later life.

An annual pelvic examination is the best protection against cancer of the ovary.

### What about hormones and cervical cancer?

Recent evidence suggests that there is an increased incidence of cervical tumors in women who are on long-term oral contraceptives. No data are available for women on postmenopausal hormone replacement therapy (HRT).

Since precancerous changes in the cervix can be spotted with a Pap smear many years before the cancer develops, a yearly Pap smear is the best protection. Women at high risk for cervical cancer are those who had their first sexual intercourse before the age of 17, who have had more than three sexual partners, or who smoke.

### What about hormones and breast cancer?

One out of every 10 newborn females will develop breast cancer during her life. The leading cause of death in women age 40-44 is breast cancer. The risk of breast cancer continues to increase with age: the chance of developing breast cancer is six times greater at the age of 70 than at the age of 40. The statistics go on and on.

Although two early studies reported increased risk of breast cancer with hormone therapy, multiple, large, long-term studies how conclusively show that the rate of breast cancer is not greater for women using birth control pills or postmenopausal hormones.

The report by R. Don Gambrell, Jr., M.D., published in the October 1984 issue of *Current Problems in Obstetrics and Gynecology*, heralds a significant change in thinking about hormones in women with estrogen and progesterone deficiencies. This study corroborates previous studies indicating that estrogen replacement therapy does not increase the incidence of breast cancer even in those groups at high risk for it. In addition, it shows that long-term use of cyclic progesterone actually decreases the risk of breast cancer. Figure 11 illustrates the results of this study.

The incidence of breast cancer in users of cyclic estrogen-progesterone was 67 cases per 100,000 women. This is significantly lower than the incidence of breast cancer in this age group according to the Third National

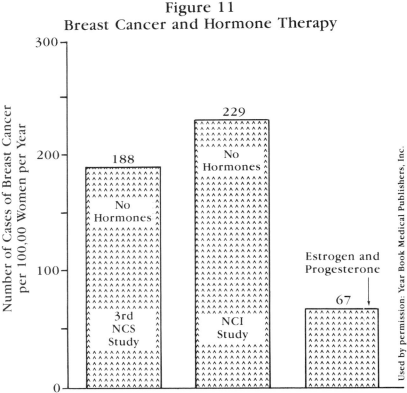

Figure 11
Breast Cancer and Hormone Therapy

Note: 3rd NCS = National Cancer Survey Study
NCI = National Cancer Institute Study

Cancer Survey, which finds 188 cases per 100,000 women. It is also significantly lower than the incidence according to the National Cancer Institute SEER data, which list 229 cases per 100,000 women.

This study suggests that progesterone must be used over some time before it shows a protective effect on the breast. In the study, it appears that the effect of the cyclic progesterone is not significantly apparent until it has been used for at least four years. This goes along with the basic science studies showing that the number of estrogen receptor sites in the breast is positively correlated with an increased risk of breast cancer. Cyclic use of progesterone causes a decrease in the number of these estrogen receptor sites. However, these basic science studies have shown that obtaining the decrease requires long-term use of progesterone.

This finding of a decrease in the risk of breast cancer in postmenopausal women who take cyclic progesterone has prompted many physicians to treat their post-hysterectomy patients with cyclic progesterone even though they do not need the progesterone for cyclic emptying of the uterus. Unfortunately, as discussed under other questions, progesterone may partially or completely reverse the beneficial effects of estrogen on the risk of heart disease.

The use of progesterone for protection against breast cancer is still a controversial issue. The issue of the use of progesterone in hormone replacement therapy is discussed in greater detail under the question "What is considered the best hormone replacement therapy for the postmenopausal woman?" in Chapter 5.

In coming years, we can expect much more information concerning this apparent protection from breast cancer.

# 5
# HORMONE REPLACEMENT THERAPY

## When should hormone replacement therapy (HRT) start?

With regard to hormonal production, a woman's life has four important time periods:

- *First period:* From birth to the first menses (menarche)
- *Second period:* From menarche, through the child-bearing years, to the time when the woman begins to experience symptoms of the approaching menopause
- *Third period:* From the start of the symptoms of the approaching menopause (menstrual irregularities, hot flashes, and mood swings) to the actual time of the menopause
- *Fourth period:* From the last menstrual period (menopause), continuing through the remainder of the woman's life (postmenopause)

Hormone therapy can be used during all four periods of a woman's life. In the first hormonal period, a physician

59

may prescribe estrogen creams applied locally to the genitalia of girls to treat irritations and to release the lips of the vaginal opening when they are fused.

Physicians frequently prescribe hormones during the second hormonal period of a woman's life. They are used for treatment of infertility; for control of heavy, irregular, and/or prolonged periods; and last, but far from least, for birth control.

For women who are in the third portion of their hormonal life and who experience the premenopausal symptoms of menstrual irregularities, hot flashes, and mood swings, hormone therapy may be very effective. There is evidence that hormonal treatment of these symptoms can also have some long-term benefits: strengthening a woman's bones, protection against cardiovascular disease, and reducing her risk of uterine cancer.

Hormone replacement therapy (HRT) is critically important to the woman in the fourth hormonal period of her life. There is some controversy among physicians as to when or (in some cases) if HRT should be started. I strongly disagree with any physician who states that, in general, women do not need HRT or should start HRT only when it has been proved that degenerative changes are taking place.

The entire first part of this book should have convinced you that, except in cases where hormone use is definitely inadvisable, women will benefit from the use of HRT in the postmenopausal period of life.

As discussed earlier, osteoporosis is a debilitating disease found in many postmenopausal women. For various reasons, not all postmenopausal women experience the degenerative effects of osteoporosis at the same rate. Estrogen therapy can stop, and to some extent correct, postmenopausal osteoporosis. The problem therefore is whether to start the HRT only after finding laboratory or symptomatic signs of osteoporosis, or to start HRT before the disease develops.

"Early" HRT therapy is started while the woman is still having symptoms of the perimenopause, such as hot flashes, depression, anxiety, or infrequent periods. This is when all women should start HRT. It is well documented that when a woman allows herself to go through the menopause and into the postmenopause without HRT, she allows irreversible changes to occur. These changes have an especially detrimental effect on her bones and blood vessels.

Tests for the development of osteoporosis are available. However, they are expensive, and by the time the diagnosis of osteoporosis is made, significant amounts of irreplaceable bone have been lost. Starting therapy after osteoporosis has been diagnosed is *too late*. Remember the old adage, "It is too late to close the barn door after the horses have gotten away." Calcium lost from the bones during the early years of the menopause is not replaceable with any known therapy, including high doses of calcium or HRT. Most physicians who believe in HRT agree that it should be started with the first definite symptom of the menopause.

Some studies are beginning to suggest that in certain women osteoporosis may begin well before the time of the last menses (menopause) and that the loss of bone is due in part to decreased levels of estrogen before the actual menopause. Future studies may show that complete HRT before the cessation of all menses may be valuable in protecting a woman's bones.

### What about HRT for menstrual irregularities that occur just before the menopause?

The third time period of a woman's hormonal life was defined in the preceding question. During this time, the ovaries contain few eggs and are prone to function erratically. One of the first aggravating symptoms to show up is irregularity in the menses. The woman may experience more frequent periods, or skipped periods, as well as heavy and prolonged flow. A woman who had regular, 28-day cycles all her life may find that she is having cycles that vary from 14 to 56 or more days. Instead of having the usual five to seven days of bleeding, she may have three to five days of spotting, then several days of flow, some of which may be very heavy with clots, and finally another three to five days of spotting. Another common possibility is seven to ten days of flow, of which several days are so heavy with clotting that she finds it difficult to protect herself.

If the woman ignores these changes, she will often become very tired and rundown, especially after a heavy period. The fatigue is usually caused by the development of anemia. I never cease to be amazed at finding a hemoglobin (the measuring of anemia) of 7 or 8 grams in patients showing up in my office complaining of persistent heavy periods; the normal hemoglobin in a healthy woman should be 13 to 14 grams.

The problem in these women is that the number of eggs remaining in their ovaries is so low that they frequently do not produce an egg. During a cycle without ovulation, estrogen is produced but irregularly and usually in small amounts. Because the estrogen rapidly drops to a very low level before the menses, the woman commonly begins to experience hot flashes just before or during her menses. Spotting can occur before the menstrual flow because of erratic, low levels of estrogen production.

In addition, during cycles where no ovulation takes place, no progesterone is produced. This leaves the uterine lining "unripened," that is, not ready to be shed from the uterine walls. The time between periods may also be much longer than usual, causing prolonged estrogen stimulation and thereby excessive growth of the uterine lining. These two factors—unripened lining and overstimulated lining—will lead to extremely heavy flow and clotting. See "What is the menstrual cycle?" (Chapter 1) and "What are the most common early signs of the menopause?" (Chapter 2).

The appropriate use of estrogen and progesterone in this third period of a woman's hormonal life could possibly relieve some of these aggravating symptoms. Use of progesterone for 10 days starting on the 16th day of the cycle frequently corrects the irregular and heavy periods. (Physicians number the days of a menstrual cycle from the first day of flow. Therefore, the 16th day of the cycle means 16 days from the first day of the menstrual flow.)

The progesterone has two effects. First, it causes ripening of the uterine lining, which estrogen has stimulated to grow. Second, stopping the progesterone after 10 days causes the uterine lining to die and slough off: a period occurs. If a woman with irregular and/or heavy periods uses the 10 days of progesterone for every cycle, she will have regular periods that are usually shorter and lighter. Use of progesterone in this way stops excessive growth of uterine lining and ripens the uterine lining, allowing a normal menses. Most physicians refer to this method as "terminal progesterone therapy" (see Appendix C).

When a woman with menstrual irregularities seeks the aid of her physician, the doctor may handle her in several ways. If the patient has had heavy and irregular periods, without bleeding between the periods, and is 45 or younger, the doctor may elect to start her on the cyclic progesterone. If, however, the patient is having an extremely heavy period at the time, the doctor will frequently suggest one of two methods for rapid control of the heavy bleeding occurring at the time. One method is surgical, and the other is nonsurgical.

The surgical approach is a D&C (dilatation and curettage). This is a minor surgical procedure, usually performed in an outpatient facility. The uterus is scraped out while the patient is under general anesthesia. This procedure quickly and effectively empties the uterus and controls the bleeding. Subsequent pain is minimal. Mild cramping may be present, but it seldom requires pain medication. Complications of the surgery are rare. The woman can expect to return to her regular activities within 24 to 48 hours.

This procedure not only stops the bleeding quickly, but it also allows the physician to determine the cause of the bleeding, and in certain cases it corrects the problem. Although hormonal changes are the most common cause of this kind of bleeding, there are other causes. The presence of fibroid tumors, endometrial polyps, or a condition known as adenomyosis can also cause excessively heavy and prolonged periods. These conditions are more fully described in Appendix B.

The nonsurgical approach to the problem of heavy menstrual bleeding is the use of birth control pills. Some physicians simply prescribe birth control pills to be taken in the usual "one a day" pattern for a few cycles. I have found that giving a patient a package of 21 pills and having her take five immediately, four the next day, three the next, two the next, and one per day thereafter until they are gone, is a more effective and rapid method of controlling heavy bleeding. This method will usually override whatever abnormal hormonal cycle is going on in the patient, bring all the lining to a ripened stage, and, after the pills are finished, cause a menses that allows complete emptying of the uterine cavity. Among physicians, this method is frequently referred to as a "medical D&C."

Use of birth control pills in this way poses no danger to the woman, no matter what her age, unless she has already had a significant problem (side effect) with the Pill. Some physicians prefer to use decreasing doses of progesterone alone for this kind of problem; however, in my experience, progesterone alone has not been nearly as effective as birth control pills.

The use of terminal progesterone therapy in women having heavy, prolonged, and irregular periods is a common, accepted practice by most physicians. Besides regulating the cycle and lightening the flow, this therapy has an important hidden advantage. As discussed under the question "What about hormones and uterine cancer?" (Chapter 4), we know that prolonged and repeated stimulation of the uterine lining without cyclic progesterone can lead to overstimulated cells and possibly to development of a cancer of the uterine lining. Cyclic use of 10 days of progesterone prevents this overstimulation of the uterine lining cells. This cancer avoidance is a very important benefit. See Appendix C for information about terminal progesterone therapy in young women with infrequent and/or irregular periods.

Some women experience uncomfortable hot flashes at various times during their cycle. This occurs when the estrogen drops below a level the woman can tolerate without having symptoms. Drops like this can occur at the time of ovulation, when the egg coming out of the egg cyst disrupts the function of the egg cyst. When estrogen production is already at a critically low level, as it is for women close to the menopause, the drop in estrogen production can cause midcycle hot flashes as well as spotting. Just before the menses, the estrogen level can again fall below a critical level and remain there for most of the menses, causing the woman to have hot flashes.

This drop in estrogen can also cause other symptoms during the menses that the patient has not experienced in previous years. These symptoms include headaches, lethargy, and insomnia. Use of a low dose of estrogen (Premarin, 0.3 milligram per day) during the midcycle and just before and during the menses often can alleviate these symptoms.

Once a woman has reached this third part of her hormonal life and has started terminal progesterone therapy to alleviate her symptoms, she should remain on it until she no longer has a period after taking the ten days of progesterone. Some women decide before they truly reach the menopause that they don't need the progesterone. They stop the medication and may continue to have regular normal periods. This leads them to believe that they were correct and no longer need the medication. However, the approach of menopause is unrelenting, just like the IRS. The symptoms will recur in time, when they may be more severe, ending in severe bleeding or a uterine cancer. The closer you are to the age of menopause (the average age of menopause in the United States is 51.4 years), the more definitely you should stay on terminal progesterone therapy once you have started it.

When you no longer respond to the progesterone with a period, you have reached the true menopause and are no longer producing enough estrogen to stimulate the uterine lining to grow. At this time, you should start total hormonal replacement therapy (HRT), if you have not already done so. Most women would have experienced significantly increased hot flashes by this time and would have requested additional therapy. With the occurrence of the true menopause, you have entered the fourth period of your hormonal life, the postmenopause, and should remain on full HRT from then on.

### What is considered the best hormone replacement therapy for the postmenopausal woman?

Historically, intramuscular injections of animal-extracted estrogen were used to treat the symptoms of the perimenopause. Most of these preparations were long-acting medications. Effective control of menopausal symptoms lasted three to six weeks. Women usually received monthly injections. As already discussed under the question "What about hormones and uterine cancer?" (Chapter 4), the problems with this kind of therapy are that the estrogen is continuous, is unopposed by cyclic progesterone, and does not allow the uterus to completely empty its growth of uterine lining at the time of menses. This all adds up to an increased risk of cancer.

In 1938, the first oral synthetic estrogen compound, diethylstilbestrol (DES), was produced. It was eventually used for treatment of menopausal symptoms, as well as for women who were threatening to miscarry. This latter use has been greatly publicized in relation to the increased risk of vaginal tumors in the daughters of women who were treated with the drug. However, that's an entirely different story, which we need not get into in this book. The mothers who took the drug have not experienced any increase in the rate of vaginal cancers.

Shortly thereafter, conjugated estrogens, extracted from pregnant mares, were developed and sold for the treatment of perimenopausal symptoms. Up until the 1960s, these drugs were used as continuous daily therapy or on a cycle of 21 days on and 7 days off. This type of unopposed estrogen therapy, as expected, led to an increased risk of endometrial cancer.

In 1960 the oral progesterones became available, but their use in menopausal therapy was suggested by only a few researchers. At that early date, some even suggested that use of cyclic progesterone might be of value in protecting against endometrial cancer. However, whereas the use of estrogens for treatment of menopausal symptoms rapidly became popular, the additional use of progesterone did not gain the same popularity.

In the 1970s, three independent studies reported a 4-14 percent increase in uterine cancer in women who took estrogen for more than one year. The FDA jumped in with the patient-warning inserts that must be given to each patient receiving a prescription of estrogen. The FDA statement is reprinted in Appendix A.

It wasn't until 1978 that the use of cyclic progesterone along with estrogen really caught on in the medical profession. Since that time, a number of studies have shown the importance of using progesterone in menopausal hormone replacement therapy (HRT). As already discussed under the question "What about hormones and uterine cancer?" (Chapter 4), these studies showed that when progesterone is used in conjunction with estrogen, not only is there no increase in the rate of uterine cancer, but the rate actually decreases.

Most internists and gynecologists agree that the combination of cyclic estrogen and progesterone is not only the most effective, but also the most advantageous type of therapy. My personal preference is the use of estrogen from the 1st through the 25th day of each month. To this I add a progesterone from the 16th through the 25th day of each month. The patient does not take any hormones from the 26th until the 1st of the next month. The doses of estrogen and progesterone vary from patient to patient and from product to product.

There is conclusive evidence that estrogens protect the postmenopausal women against osteoporosis; thinning of the supportive tissues of the skin, vagina, and bladder; hot flashes; and the other bothersome symptoms of the menopause syndrome. Estrogens also reduce the risk of heart disease. Use of estrogen alone increases the risk of uterine cancer, while the addition of progesterone not only corrects that increased risk but seems to decrease the rate of uterine cancer by 50 percent in women who use it along with their cyclic estrogen. The great majority of authorities on this subject agree with all the statements in this paragraph.

Some physicians, however, are less convinced about the use of cyclic progesterone. The answer to "What about hormones and breast cancer?" (Chapter 4) discussed the recent studies of Dr. Gambrell concerning a significant decrease in the rate of breast cancer in women who used cyclic progesterone for longer than four years. However, these findings are not fully accepted by the medical community. If they should prove to be correct, then there is *no doubt* that the "best" regimen for hormonal therapy must include cyclic progesterone.

For the sake of this discussion, assume that this protection against breast cancer by progesterone proves to be incorrect. At the onset of menopause, a white female living in the United States has a 0.5 percent risk of dying from uterine cancer during the remainder of her life. This is in contrast to at least a ten times greater risk of dying from heart attack related to atherosclerosis. As discussed earlier, estrogen replacement therapy given in the menopause reduces the risk of fatal and nonfatal atherogenic heart disease by 50 percent. This is due, in part, to estrogen's ability to lower the low-density lipoproteins and elevate the high-density lipoproteins in the blood. The addition of a progesterone seems to reverse this process to some degree. Progesterones, therefore, may decrease the protection against heart disease.

With this in mind, some physicians feel that until we have more evidence showing that progesterones truly do protect against breast cancer or that cyclic progesterones do not increase the risk of heart disease, women should not use progesterones if they no longer have a uterus and therefore are not at risk of developing uterine cancer because of overstimulation by receiving estrogen alone. Some even go further and say that in women with an intact functioning uterus, the protection a woman gets from atherosclerotic heart disease by taking estrogen alone far outweighs the risk of death from a uterine cancer stimulated by estrogen alone. They therefore suggest that women not use cyclic progesterone for protection against uterine cancer.

It certainly would be tragic if we lost one of the major benefits of estrogen in terms of atherosclerotic heart disease by using progesterone. Medroxyprogesterone (Provera) does not seem to reduce high-density lipoproteins (HDL) significantly, but present-day studies are in conflict concerning this point. As of this time, we lack sufficient data to determine the long-term effect of progesterone on heart disease. By monitoring my patients' HDL cholesterol levels, I can offer them the best of both estrogen and progesterone therapy with safety. In my patients on cyclic estrogen-progesterone therapy, I have not found any significant decrease in HDL.

In addition, if women used estrogen alone from the onset of menopause, the necessity of yearly endometrial biopsies, the occurrence of irregular spotting or heavy prolonged irregular bleeding, and the fear of developing a uterine cancer might cause them to avoid taking the medication and even stop the estrogen therapy altogether. Although there is controversy regarding the use of progesterone with postmenopausal estrogen therapy, cyclic estrogen-progesterone therapy as described in the last question is of value for the patient's overall comfort and compliance. If research eventually substantiates the role of progesterone in protecting against breast cancer, then there will be no doubt about the routine use of progesterone in hormonal replacement therapy.

The types of estrogen and progesterone preparations available, suggested dosages, and variations in their use are discussed in the next few questions.

### *Is there more than one estrogen hormone?*

*Estrogen* refers to a broad category of chemical compounds that affect the female organs, including the breasts, vulva, vagina, uterus, fallopian tubes, and ovaries. These compounds also affect bone, skin, bladder, blood vessels, and hormone-producing glands, as already alluded to in prior questions. The term *estrogen* can refer to a natural or synthetic compound.

In humans, there are principally three natural estrogenic hormones: (1) estradiol; (2) estrone; and (3) estriol. Of these three estrogens, estradiol is the most potent and the major product secreted by the ovaries. During the normal menstrual cycle, estradiol is synthesized by the developing follicle (egg cyst). The rate of secretion of estradiol varies widely during the cycle. Estradiol is the main stimulus to activity in target organs.

Estradiol can be easily chemically transformed to the less potent estrone; however, estrone is mainly produced by a second process outside of the ovary. This process is termed *extraglandular production*. Because extraglandular production is not cyclic, the rate of estrone formation does not vary appreciably during the menstrual cycle. Figure 12 compares the fluctuating levels of estradiol produced by the developing egg follicle to the more constant lower levels of estrone produced outside the ovary.

Estriol is considered to have the weakest estrogenic properties of the three kinds of estrogen. It is considered

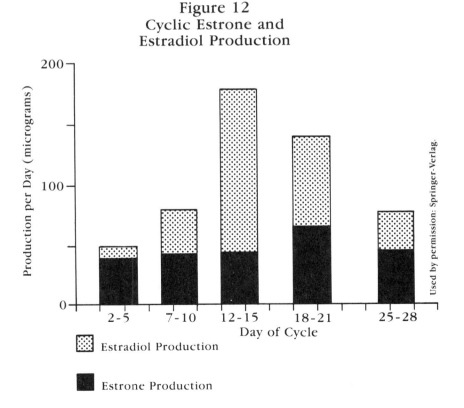

## Figure 12
## Cyclic Estrone and
## Estradiol Production

to be mainly a metabolic product of estradiol and estrone. At the present time, estriol is neither readily available nor frequently used in hormone replacement therapy.

The synthesis, metabolism, and excretion of these three estrogens are complex. A description of these biochemical and physiological reactions is beyond the scope of this book.

The fact that the natural estrogens are virtually insoluble in water greatly limits their absorption from the stomach or intestines. The effectiveness of orally administered natural estrogens is further limited because it requires transformation while the body absorbs it from the intestine and while it passes through the liver. Most orally administered "natural" estradiol is transformed to estrone in the stomach and enters the blood as estrone. The small amount of estradiol that the body directly absorbs from the intestines is further processed and inactivated as it passes through the liver before reaching the bloodstream.

Manufacturers of estrogenic hormones have tried various methods to improve the intestinal absorption of these estrogens. One that has been found to improve the absorption of orally administered estradiol is "micronization." This method is used to produce a product known as Estrace. The process involves reducing the particle size of the natural estradiol so that more of it can be absorbed. Micronization has been shown to increase the blood levels of active estradiol and estrone above those of identical doses of nonmicronized, orally administered estradiol.

As mentioned, estrone in its natural state is relatively insoluble in water and therefore is poorly absorbed from the intestines. However, changing it by chemical processes called conjugation or esterification improves its solubility and makes it effective when taken orally. One such group of commercially available estrones are called "conjugated estrogens."

Conjugated estrogens are one of the earliest commercially available estrogenic compounds used for HRT. Premarin is a popular, commercially available conjugated estrogen product. It is probably the most commonly prescribed estrogen for HRT. Premarin is prepared from the urine of pregnant mares. This naturally occurring estrogenic compound is made up of 70-percent sodium estrone sulfate and 20-percent equilenin sulfate. The remaining 10 percent of estrogenic compounds are small amounts of other equine (horse) by-products, which are thought to be of little significance. The sodium estrone sulfate and equilenin sulfate are readily absorbed from the intestines, and the blood level of equilenin in a person who takes conjugated estrogens actually exceeds the blood level of estradiol. The significance of these levels of equilenin in the human is unknown and has not been shown to be of concern.

Equilenin is excreted from the bloodstream very slowly. Significant levels of this equine estrogen have been found in women three months after they discontinue Premarin therapy. However, increasing blood levels of equilenin, above those achieved with initial treatment, have not been shown to occur with extended use of Premarin. At the present state of our knowledge, the presence of equilenin in Premarin and other conjugated estrogen preparations give no particular advantage or disadvantage compared to other preparations.

Most of the research done with conjugated estrogens has been done with Premarin. This is especially true with respect to HRT. Generic conjugated estrogens and so-called esterified equine estrogens (Menest) are mixtures of naturally occurring estrogenic compounds. The percentages of estrone, equilenin, and other equine compounds may vary as much as 20 percent. Neither the FDA nor the manufacturers of generic conjugated estrogens can assure us that the generic conjugated or esterified equine estrogens have the equivalent effectiveness of the Premarin. Because I have encountered problems in my patients who used generic estrogens, I prescribe Premarin rather than the generic conjugated estrogens.

The process called esterification changes the insoluble natural estrone to a sulfate ester, which is a more soluble form. Ogen is one of the more popular commercial preparations in this group. Treatment with Ogen is basically treatment with estrone alone. The estrogenic potency seems to be less when compared milligram for milligram with Premarin. However, in many patients, equal doses of Ogen and Premarin give the same subjective results. One final comment concerning Ogen: some research data show that Ogen may have less effect of increasing blood pressure than conjugated estrogens have, although this is not a universally accepted fact and the studies that developed the data have been challenged.

To summarize, the major groups of commercially available estrogenic hormones considered to be natural are micronized estradiol (Estrace), conjugated estrogens (Premarin or generic), esterified estrogens (Menest or generic), and sulfate esters of estrone (Ogen). All of these products, when taken orally, cause increases in the blood levels of estradiol and estrone, as well as smaller quantities of various other estrogenic compounds. One unresolved problem with all these products is the development of abnormal ratios of estrone to estradiol in the blood.

In a normal menstruating (premenopausal) woman, the ratio of estrone to estradiol is usually less than 1:1. In a postmenopausal woman not taking HRT, the ratio is usually 2-4:1. When any of the natural estrogen products are used for oral HRT, the estrone/estradiol ratios are increased to 3-6:1. The significance of this ratio remains unknown. Since any one of these estrogenic hormones can be rapidly transformed into any other estrogenic hormone, the estrone/estradiol ratio may not really be critical. A woman's body may quickly change whatever basic estrogenic compound it gets into whatever compound it needs.

Some work has been done with other ways to administer hormones. Vaginal administration of micronized estradiol is more effective than the oral route. Smaller doses achieve higher blood levels. In addition, absorption from the vagina bypasses the liver, leading to a lower and more natural ratio of estrone to estradiol. Other routes for administering hormones are being studied, including nose drops, tablets placed under the tongue, shots, and administration through skin patches. At the present time, the oral route of estrogen therapy is the only route that effectively relieves hot flashes; atrophy of bladder, vagina, and skin; osteoporosis; and atherosclerosis. (See Appendix D for additional information on administration through skin patches.) Until new products or new modes of administration of estrogenic compounds are found, we will have to accept the problems of excessive estrone/estradiol blood levels in order to attain sufficient levels of estradiol to relieve menopausal symptoms.

Injectable, long-acting estradiol is available for use in postmenopausal women. The safety of long-term use of this type of preparation is still subject to considerable debate. This route of administration seems to lead to higher ratios of estrone to estradiol and, in general, causes these substances to remain longer in the blood at peak levels. Some evidence suggests that prolonged use of this method may increase unwanted vaginal bleeding, heavy and prolonged menstruation, and possibly breast cancer. Present knowledge suggests that injectable, long-acting estrogenic compounds should be used only over short periods of time (one to two years). In those unusual cases where long-term therapy is found necessary, women should be warned about the unknown dangers and receive close follow-up care.

In addition to the "natural" estrogens, there are purely synthetic estrogenic compounds. They are capable of producing all the responses of natural estrogens.

Diethylstilbestrol (DES) was first isolated in 1938. Later that year, a second compound, ethinyl estradiol, was synthesized. DES is rapidly and completely absorbed from the intestine, and it has a prolonged excretion time, causing blood levels to persist for two or three days. Ethinyl estradiol is also rapidly and completely absorbed from the intestines. It is commercially available in doses ranging from 0.01 to 0.5 milligram. It is roughly 25 times as potent as diethylstilbestrol. Mestranol, a chemical variant of ethinyl estradiol, is nearly as potent estrogenically and is also widely used in oral contraceptives. Some of the early osteoporosis studies showed that these synthetic estrogens protected against bone loss arising from estrogen deficiency. All of the above synthetic estrogens are seldom, if ever, used for HRT.

Quinestrol is a synthetic that is absorbed from the intestine, stored in the body fat, and slowly released into the bloodstream. It is commercially available as Estrovis. It is initially taken once a day for one week. This loads the body fat. It is then taken once a week as a maintenance dose. Adequate data do not exist to establish that quinestrol has a positive effect on any but the subjective symptoms of the menopause (such as hot flashes, insomnia, and depression). Research has not established whether it offers adequate protection to the bones, supportive tissues, and the cardiovascular system. Further, it does not offer the important menstrual cycling factor that is necessary in women with an intact uterus. For post-hysterectomy women, Estrovis is certainly convenient with its weekly dosage. When the uterus is absent, cyclic progesterone, for the supposed breast cancer protection, can be used for 10 consecutive days each month along with the weekly Estrovis.

No studies prove or disprove that this drug and method of administration protect the bones, blood vessels, or connective tissues as does a cyclic daily dose of short-acting estrogens. Further, women using this compound may find it necessary to take it every three to six days in order to keep themselves free of hot flashes and other subjective symptoms.

At this time, it is premature to condemn or praise the use of any of the commercially available compounds described beyond the comments made here. As research continues, the "best" compounds may become obvious.

### How does the potency of commercially available estrogen preparations compare?

One of the major problems concerning HRT is the lack of good comparative studies concerning the potency, effects, and side effects of the various commercially available preparations. We can compare the potency of these compounds in several ways. For instance, we can look at how well an estrogenic preparation controls subjective symptoms such as hot flashes, depression, or insomnia. More scientifically, we can look at the objective effects.

The subjective symptoms—hot flashes, depression, irritability, fatigue, and so on—are hard to use in measuring potency because the response varies so much from one person to another. Because all of these symptoms can arise from conditions other than estrogen deficiency, the complexity of sorting out the various causes is so involved that measuring a product's effect on them is difficult and unreliable.

The effect of these preparations on subjective symptoms is best determined for each individual patient, by trial and effect. Because the objective effects of these drugs on the body are measurable, this is a valuable way to compare their potency.

One objective way to measure the potency of an estrogenic substance is to see how well is suppresses the hormones called pituitary gonadotropins. These hormones are more prevalent in estrogen-deficient postmenopausal women. Suppressing them is considered a "good effect," since it lowers gonadotropin levels to those found in the premenopausal woman and indicates that activity of the pituitary gland is reduced to normal.

Another objective way to measure potency of estrogens

is to assess the effect of oral estrogen preparations on stimulating the liver to produce certain compounds. One such compound is angiotensin, which can increase the blood pressure. Although the total significance of stimulating liver metabolism is not fully understood, it is thought to be an undesirable effect of estrogen therapy.

It is difficult to know which of the various measures are the most important to the user's health. This discussion uses the objective parameters described to compare the potency of the various commercially available preparations.

Gonadotropin suppression can be measured objectively and is considered a desirable effect. The drug piperazine esterified estrone (Ogen) has the least relative effectiveness in suppressing the elevated level of pituitary gonadotropin in the menopausal woman's blood. Micronized estradiol (Estrace) and conjugated estrogens (Premarin) are slightly more effective in suppressing these gonadotropin levels. For all practical purposes, the 1.25-milligram dose of Ogen is equal to the 1-milligram dose of Estrace and the 0.9-milligram dose of Premarin in respect to this measure. DES and ethinyl estradiol (Estinyl), two of the synthetic estrogenic preparations, are far more potent than the natural estrogens. A dose of 0.5 milligram of DES or 0.01 milligram of Estinyl has an equal effect in decreasing the gonadotropin levels, compared to 1 milligram of the natural preparation.

These five types of estrogenic substances are remarkably different in the degree to which they stimulate the liver. Ogen and Estrace have little effect on liver metabolism when given in doses up to 1.25 milligrams and 1 milligram, respectively. However, doses of Premarin at or above 0.625 milligram significantly stimulate the liver. This stimulation may result from the high and persistent levels of the equine estrogen, equilenin. Significant stimulation occurs with even the smallest doses of DES (0.1 milligram) and Estinyl (0.01 milligram). This exaggerated response suggests—but does not prove—that the synthetic preparations are less desirable preparations for HRT.

Little conclusive evidence exists to show any significant differences in potency, effects, or side effects of the natural estrogen products (conjugated estrogens, estrone sulfate esters, micronized estradiol, esterified estrogens). I therefore cannot, with clear conscience, suggest one over another.

The manufacturers of micronized estradiol (Estrace), esterified estrogens (Menest), and estrone sulfate esters (Ogen) would like us to believe that their products are superior to the conjugated estrogens (Premarin and generic) because those products contain horse estrogen impurities. They also would point out that blood levels obtained from a dose of conjugated estrogens is higher for the equine estrogen equilenin than for the human estrogens estrone or estradiol. However, no one has been able to show that this high, prolonged level of equilenin has any deleterious effects in a woman.

Some studies indicate that conjugated estrogens are more apt to raise blood pressure, as mentioned in relation to their tendency to stimulate liver metabolism. But adequate scientific information is not yet available for making a definitive decision concerning the effect of conjugated estrogens on blood pressure.

One of the major attributes of conjugated estrogens, especially Premarin, is that they have been used for HRT far more extensively and longer than any of the other estrogens. Most of the scientific studies showing the benefits of estrogen on the body have been done with conjugated estrogens. With this vast, long-term experience, no scientific study has to my knowledge been able to prove beyond doubt that any of the other estrogen preparations are better for HRT. Premarin is also the least expensive of these products.

I prescribe Premarin, Estrace, and Ogen, in that order among my patients. I change products, based on the patient's response. Where one patient may not like Premarin for one subjective reason or another, she may get along just fine on Ogen or Estrace. At the same time, another patient may prefer Estrace over the others for the same reason someone else preferred Premarin.

### Is there more than one progesterone hormone?

The term *progesterone* refers to a specific organic chemical compound and therefore is different from the term *estrogen*, which refers to a group of chemical compounds that are related by their similar biologic activity. Progesterone is secreted by the ovaries. More specifically, it is a product of the lutein cells of the functioning corpus luteum cyst. The term *progesterones* is sometimes used to indicate synthetic products which have effects similar to the hormone progesterone. However, the correct term for these synthetic products is *progestins,* or *progestogens.*

As you will recall from the description in answer to the question "What is the menstrual cycle?" (Chapter 1), the egg develops in the ovary in a small cyst called the follicle cyst. The cells of this cyst (follicle cells) produce increasing amounts of estrogen. When ovulation occurs, the follicle cyst breaks open, expelling the egg into the abdominal cavity or fallopian tube. The cyst then collapses, and a change in the cellular structure of the cyst occurs; lutein cells develop. These lutein cells continue to produce estrogen but also begin to produce increasing amounts of progesterone.

Progesterone's main effect is on the uterine lining, or endometrium. It causes the endometrium to prepare for implantation of a fertilized egg, should one be available. The only other known major effect of progesterone is on the breasts. During pregnancy, progesterone causes the breasts to prepare for lactation (production of milk).

Progesterone has another important effect on the menstruating woman. Mineral balance and water storage change cyclically with menstruation. These changes come about because progesterone acts upon the kidneys to prevent loss of water, sodium, and chloride, while it speeds the loss of potassium. The water content also increases in the cerebral cortex of the brain, tending to produce a temporary lack of blood in the surrounding tissues.

This could explain the development of premenstrual tension syndrome (PMS) before and during menstruation, which is characterized by increased sensitivity, irritability, water retention, uterine cramps, and breast tenderness. Paradoxically, when large amounts of progesterone are given to women, the hormone has a sedative effect on the central nervous system and on uterine activity. This may account for the success of a modern therapy for PMS: a large dose of progesterone starting several days before the period.

### What progesterone preparations are commercially available?

Naturally occurring progesterone taken orally is not absorbed to any significant extent. It is rapidly absorbed when dissolved in oil and given by injection into the muscles. However, the action of progesterone given in this manner is short-lived. To use progesterone for HRT in this form, the patient would have to get daily shots for at least 10 days each month.

Natural progesterone in oil can be placed into capsules or suppositories for use in the vagina. Absorption from the vagina is very good. I have prescribed vaginal applications of 100 to 400 milligrams of progesterone daily for 5-10 days before menses to effectively control premenstrual tension syndrome (PMS). In most cases, however, women receiving HRT for menopausal symptoms would rather not use a vaginal application.

Some progesterone preparations, such as Delalutin and Depoprovera, are long-acting medications injected into the muscles. However, their absorption and duration of action are not consistent. They therefore have little practical use in postmenopausal HRT.

For use in HRT, there are basically two groups of oral synthetic progesterones (progestins) available on the market. Medroxyprogesterone acetate (Provera) is a derivative of progesterone. Surprisingly, even though it is insoluble in water, it is effectively absorbed from the digestive tract. The second group of progesterones is made up of derivatives of testosterone or, more precisely, 19-nor-testosterone, a major male hormone. Basically two compounds in this group are available for HRT. They are norethindrone (Norlutin) and norethindrone acetate (Aygestin and Norlutate), and they differ only in potency. The acetate is approximately twice as potent. Another testosterone derivative is norgestrel, which is 100 times more potent as a progesterone than norethindrone. It is used mainly in oral contraceptives and is not available alone for HRT.

Using estrogen therapy to prevent bone loss in postmenopausal women has already been discussed under the question "How can postmenopausal osteoporosis be prevented or treated?" (Chapter 3). Some evidence suggests that progesterone therapy also may be effective in preventing osteoporosis. As discussed in the answers to the questions about osteoporosis, estrogen therapy appears to inhibit resorption of calcium, thereby halting the loss of minerals from the bone. Although studies have not shown that estrogen therapy will replace lost mineral content, some evidence shows that adding progesterone to the estrogen therapy may promote formation of new bone tissue. It appears important to begin the estrogen-progesterone therapy soon after the menopause. If it is started more than three years afterward, further bone loss is delayed, but bone mineral content does not increase.

The possible favorable effect of progesterone use on the rate of breast cancer may prove to be the most important fact favoring use of progesterone in HRT. See the discussion under the questions "What about hormones and breast cancer?" (Chapter 4) and "What is considered the best hormone replacement therapy for the postmenopausal woman?" (this chapter).

As discussed under the question "But don't birth control pills aggravate heart disease?" (Chapter 3), the menopause and the development of an estrogen-deficient state due to the decline of ovarian function leads to an increase in low-density lipoprotein (LDL) concentrations and a fall in the high-density lipoproteins (HDL). These changes lead to an increase in atherosclerosis (narrowing of the arteries) and thereby to an increase in coronary heart disease. Also, HDL in women receiving estrogen replacement therapy rises 20-30 percent. This rise in HDL seems to protect a woman's blood vessels against atherosclerosis.

When postmenopausal women undergo cyclic progestin therapy along with estrogen therapy, does the use of progestin adversely change the proportion of high- and low-density lipoproteins? Some studies have shown that changing to combined-hormone replacement therapy from estrogen-alone replacement therapy has no effect on the beneficially altered levels induced by the administration of estrogen alone. Some investigators have even suggested that adding a cyclic progestin may enhance the action of estrogen in reducing serum cholesterol.

Some evidence shows that the choice of progestin may affect HDL levels. Figure 13 shows the results of a study in which a group of women receiving replacement therapy with estrogen were, in addition, treated with one of three types of progestins. The HDL levels were elevated, as expected, by the estrogen therapy. When either of the two types of progestins derived from 19-nor-testosterone (norethindrone acetate or norgestrel) were used cyclically, the level of HDL fell to a level 20 percent below that observed with estrogen treatment alone. In contrast, the progesterone-derived preparation (Provera) did not seem to comparably reduce the level of HDL. This ad-

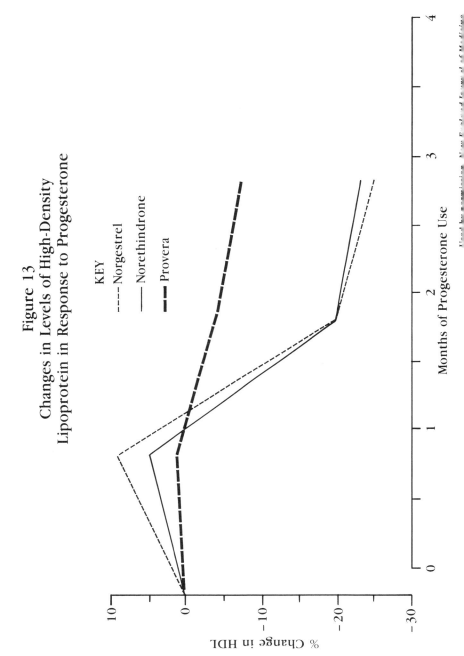

**Figure 13**
**Changes in Levels of High-Density**
**Lipoprotein in Response to Progesterone**

verse effect of the 19-nor-testosterone progestins may reflect their derivation from male hormones. It is accepted that these hormones reduce the concentration of HDL in men as well as stimulating a rise in LDL (see "What is considered the best hormone replacement therapy for the postmenopausal woman?" earlier in this chapter).

At the National Forum on Menopause Education in May 1987, Dr. Roger Lobo, M.D., an endocrinologist at the University of Southern California, reported no effect on LDL and HDL levels with use of lower doses of progestins. It is hoped that further studies will determine the most effective doses of estrogen and progesterone for maximum patient protection.

During all of a woman's premenopausal years, she enjoys a low rate of atherosclerotic heart disease. At the age of 50, a woman has 6 times less chance of having a heart attack than a man of the same age. When that woman goes through the menopause, she develops an estrogen deficiency and loses her lifelong protection against atherosclerotic disease. By the time a woman not on HRT reaches the age of 70, her chance of having a heart attack almost equals that of a 70-year-old man.

The estrogen deficiency of the untreated postmenopausal woman leads to an increase in atherosclerosis. Further, the woman has produced cyclic progesterone for most of her premenopausal life, and the progesterone she produced obviously did not neutralize the protective effect of her estrogen. It is my hope that future research will produce the knowledge necessary to find and produce estrogens and progestins that will naturally replace the hormones lost by a woman at the time of the menopause and allow her to keep all of the protective advantages she enjoyed during her premenopausal years.

The points to remember about estrogen therapy are the following:

1. Unopposed estrogen therapy (estrogen therapy without progesterone) leads to a decreased risk of atherosclerotic cardiovascular disease. (Good)
2. Unopposed estrogen therapy leads to endometrial overstimulation and thereby increases the risk of cancer of the uterine lining (endometrial cancer). (Bad)
3. The addition of progestin therapy to estrogen therapy prevents the development of overstimulation of the uterine lining and thus prevents endometrial malignancy. (Good)
4. The use of progestins along with estrogen therapy causes a potentially adverse effect on plasma lipoproteins and may cancel, to some extent, the favorable effects of estrogens on atherosclerotic cardiovascular disease. (Bad)

Based on the mixed results of combining cyclic estrogen and progesterone, this treatment may, at worst, have a neutral effect on lipoprotein and atherosclerotic vascular disease. Until this issue is resolved, a good approach where possible would be to use medroxyprogesterone (Provera) as the progesterone in HRT because of its possible decreased effect on adverse changes in lipoprotein levels. Use of the 19-nor-testosterone derivatives (Aygestin, Norlutate, Norlutin), however, should not be rejected in cases where they are advantageous. Rather than stopping HRT because of heavy periods, use of the 19-nor compounds may be helpful because they tend to produce lighter flows. Also, some women refuse the Provera because of side effects. Sometimes the use of one of the 19-nor compounds avoids these side effects. The advantages of continued use of estrogen therapy, as well as the protection from uterine cancer and possible improvement of bone mineralization from use of progestins, outweigh the possible adverse effects of the 19-nor compounds.

## How do I know if my hormone dosage is correct?

This discussion uses conjugated "natural" estrogens as a dosage standard. The various estrogen compounds available commercially were discussed earlier in this chapter under the question "How does the potency of commercially available estrogen preparations compare?"

A woman's estrogen dosage depends upon numerous factors. In women beginning therapy *at* the time of menopause, a dose of 0.625 to 1.25 milligrams or more of conjugated estrogen is usually necessary to control their symptoms. It is not important how high the dose is, but rather whether or not the woman's symptoms are controlled. Most women require 0.9 to 1.25 milligrams of conjugated estrogens in order to stop the hot flashes and other early symptoms of menopause. Fewer than 10 percent will require larger doses. However, if a woman requires larger doses, she should take them.

Women taking higher doses of estrogen than their friends should not be frightened about adverse side effects. The metabolism of one woman can be different from that of another. One woman may break down the hormones faster or excrete them faster than another. If a woman is taking doses that are excessive for her, she will experience bloating, retain water, and possibly gain weight. She may also experience early bleeding in the cycle or unusually heavy bleeding at the time of the period. The woman should bring these symptoms to the attention of her physician, who can properly adjust her estrogen dosage.

For women who have already gone through the early effects of the menopause and are no longer having periods or hot flashes, 0.625 milligram of conjugated estrogens is usually adequate for initial therapy. Medical studies have shown that 0.625 milligram of Premarin is the minimum estrogen dosage for preventing loss of calcium from bones. Smaller doses are incorrectly prescribed by some physicians. Their idea is that the smaller dose is safer and can be used continually without causing uterine bleeding, while it relieves the patient's aggravating postmenopausal symptoms.

A similar method is to use a larger dose of estrogen, such as 0.625 milligram or more, but to have the patient take it every other day or when needed for severe hot flashes or mood swings. These methods are incorrect and even dangerous. They are incorrect because they do not give the woman enough estrogen to protect her bones, although they may alleviate her hot flashes and mood swings. They are dangerous in that they cause a chronic low level of stimulation of the uterine lining. This stimulation causes the lining to grow, but since there is no cyclic progesterone, the uterus cannot rid itself of this lining. This leads to a prolonged and excessive stimulation of the same cells for months or years. In the cancer-prone patient, this overstimulation leads to development of a cancer of the uterine lining.

Doses of conjugated estrogens less than 0.625 milligram are insufficient for protecting the bones of postmenopausal women. Using less than 0.625 milligram is inadequate and poor HRT. If the woman is still experiencing hot flashes on 0.625 milligram, then the dose needs to be increased. In this type of therapy, least is not best. A woman who still has hot flashes, even though they are decreased in number or intensity, needs a larger dose of estrogen until the hot flashes stop.

On occasion, a woman may stop experiencing hot flashes but may still think she is having mood swings that she did not have before the menopause. In those cases, I would double her present dose of estrogen for one cycle. If she felt an improvement, I would stay with the higher dose.

Occasionally a patient complains either that she is unable to take enough estrogen to control her symptoms or that a dose that was adequate before is no longer working satisfactorily. Sometimes we try to blame all our problems on one thing. In this case a postmenopausal woman who has experienced hot flashes or mood swings may have other physical or psychiatric problems that are causing her similar symptoms. However, the physician and the patient may think that either the dosage is too low or the patient is not absorbing the medication as expected. Indeed, some patients seem to be unable to absorb adequate amounts of oral estrogen.

If there is a question as to whether the patient is absorbing adequate estrogen or whether the problems are other than the estrogen deficiency, it can be useful to give a patient a single shot of long-acting estrogen (effective for four to six weeks). This makes sure that the woman has truly absorbed the estrogen. If her symptoms subside, she really does need more estrogen; if they do not, then the cause of the symptoms lies elsewhere.

Various symptoms and signs indicate an estrogen dose that is too high. If a woman finds that she is having extremely heavy periods each month, lowering the estrogen dose by half may cause the periods to be lighter. Unusual weight gain on a normal or low-calorie diet and with normal physical activity may also indicate an excessive amount of estrogen. (However, progesterone is usually the culprit in weight gain.) This particular problem is sometimes difficult to identify because many women gain weight at this time of their lives. The gain is related to an actual decrease in the metabolic rate of the aging patient. It also probably is related to the gradual decrease in their everyday physical activity, as well as the tendency to eat more during sedentary activities (fishing, meetings, social lunches, watching TV, traveling, and the like). Swelling and bloating can also be a sign of excessive estrogen therapy. Finally, headaches may develop or become more frequent because of estrogen therapy. This is especially true in women who have had problems with migraine-type headaches.

With these symptoms, decreasing the dosage of estrogen may alleviate the problem. When these side effects occur, the patient should attempt to decrease her estrogen dose on a trial basis. However, she should not decrease the dose below 0.625 milligram.

If decreasing the estrogen dosage rids the woman of the unwanted side effects and keeps her satisfactorily comfortable, as far as hot flashes and subjective symptoms, then she should remain on the lower dosage. However, in some situations a woman may find that when she reaches a lower dosage and gets rid of the swelling, bloating, weight gain, or headaches, then she is again having some hot flashes or mood swings. In this case, the woman will have to give and take and decide which symptoms she would rather tolerate. Fortunately, this situation is uncommon.

In less than 5 percent of my postmenopausal patients, I find that even at doses of 0.625 milligram the patient has symptoms she cannot tolerate. In these rare cases, I either discontinue all HRT or go to the inadequate dose of 0.3 milligram, for whatever good it does. Sometimes changing the type or manufacturer of the estrogen has corrected the problem. This is certainly worth a try.

Another issue related to dosage is the effect of estrogen on blood pressure. A small group of women (probably less than 10 percent) has, or has had a tendency for, high blood pressure. The use of estrogen may aggravate this problem. Some evidence suggests that different estrogen compounds have varying effects on the blood pressure. With this in mind, if a woman finds an unusual elevation in blood pressure after starting HRT, changing the type of estrogen may alleviate this problem. See "How does the potency of commercially available estrogen preparations compare?" and Appendix D.

Progesterone dosage is also important. The progesterone dosage depends on the estrogen dose. If the woman is using 0.625 milligram of estrogen, then she should use

5 milligrams of medroxyprogesterone. When at least 1.25 milligrams of estrogen or more are used, 10 milligrams of medroxyprogesterone are used. The progesterone is usually used for 10 days. With this dose, 98 percent of the women will never have any problem with residual lining remaining in the uterus. However, 2 percent of the women will have problems of heavy or prolonged periods or spotting between periods. In those few cases, 13 days of progesterone should be used.

As previously noted, a small number of women using medroxyprogesterone (Provera) will complain of heavy periods. Use of one of the norethindrone compounds (Aygestin, Norlutate, Norlutin) will often lead to lighter periods. The pros and cons of these progesterone-like drugs are discussed under the question "Is there more than one progesterone hormone?"

### Can I start hormone replacement therapy (HRT) even many years after the menopause?

I know of no reasons why HRT cannot be started at any time in the postmenopause. Patients come in to see me who have not had a period for 15 years and who want to start hormone therapy because of what they have learned about the benefits of HRT or because they have developed severe osteoporosis and were referred by their physician specifically for HRT. Unless some conditions make HRT inadvisable, I start these women on the cyclic hormones. I have not found any unexpected problems. Many of these older women have not started having periods again.

Many of these patients make surprising comments. Although most were no longer having any hot flashes, they frequently relate to me how much better "in general" they feel. They mention an improved feeling of well-being, less tiredness, increased skin moisture, diminished arthritic aches and pains, and more energy.

## How long should I continue to take HRT?

Hormone therapy beyond the age of 74 probably offers little advantage. At that age, the rates of osteoporosis in men and women seem to be the same and are probably related to aging of the bone cells rather than any hormone deficiency. This guideline pertains only to osteoporosis.

At this time we do not know whether HRT beyond the age of 70 continues to prevent cardiovascular disease, uterine cancer, or breast cancer. There is no reason to believe that hormones do not continue to produce the same benefits that they did at younger ages. In fact, with the new preliminary information that using progesterone along with estrogen causes an increase in mineral content of bone, HRT may be beneficial to the bones of women older than 74.

At this time, I suggest to all my patients that they continue their HRT at least to the age of 74. Those who reach 74 and feel inclined to continue the therapy are encouraged to do so. Future research will doubtless clarify this question.

# 6
# EVALUATING THE
# REAL AND RUMORED
# DRAWBACKS OF HRT

*Are there risks with HRT?*

This is a difficult question with no simple answer. Everything we do involves risks. We must decide and generally are constantly deciding to do or not to do something based on the law of averages and the risk involved. Many times the risk involved is worth it, based on the advantages gained.

Medicine contains many examples of this. A woman decides to have a vaginal hysterectomy and vaginal repair in order to correct the aggravating symptoms of pelvic pressure; loss of urine when she coughs, sneezes, or strains; and possibly the protrusion of tissue from the vagina. But she knows that she risks various complications from the surgery, even death. When she elects to have the surgery, she has decided that the risk is small and the advantage gained is great and long-term. The woman who uses birth control pills decides that the risks related to taking the pills are worth it, compared to having unplanned children. In fact, many women are unaware that being pregnant and having a child is many times more dangerous, as far as losing one's life, than taking the Pill.

Some specific risks are considered to be related to ingestion of hormones, especially estrogen. Some of these have already been covered in answers to previous questions. The following list shows the risks thought to be related to HRT. Those that have not already been discussed in previous questions will be covered in the following questions.

The specific risks of hormone replacement therapy (HRT) are as follows:

• Cancer of the uterine lining
• Breast cancer
• Uterine bleeding
• Exacerbation of hypertension
• Gallstones
• Blood-clotting problems
• Alterations in metabolism of glucose (blood sugar)
• Development of tumors of the liver

Development of uterine cancer and uterine bleeding have already been discussed under the question "What about hormones and uterine cancer?" Development of breast cancer has already been discussed under the question "What about hormones and breast cancer?" Both of these questions were answered in Chapter 4.

Exacerbation of hypertension by HRT is still unresolved. Certain women seem to be more sensitive to the hormones used in HRT in that their blood pressure rises above pretherapy levels. The estrogen appears to be the troublemaker. Certain estrogen preparations seem to have more effect on the liver and the production of compounds that exacerbate hypertension than do others. This was discussed under the question "How does the potency of commercially available estrogen preparations compare?" (Chapter 5).

The incidence of increased blood pressure after institution of HRT is very low—in my experience, less than 5 percent. The advantages of HRT are so great that when high blood pressure does occur, if the blood pressure can be easily controlled with simple antihypertensive medications, it is better to take the antihypertensive medications and stay on the HRT. The benefits of the HRT probably far outweigh the inconvenience of the antihypertensive medication.

The last four risks listed will be discussed in the following questions.

## What about gallstones and HRT?

In certain women, estrogen seems to cause the bile to combine with other body salts and form stones. The incidence of gallstones in postmenopausal women using hormone replacement therapy (HRT) is 2.5 times greater than in women not using hormones. The problem is even greater in obese women. Regular gallbladder x-rays to determine which women on HRT are developing gallstones is not economically feasible.

Nevertheless, the advantages gained from use of HRT far outweigh the risks of gallstones.

## What about the risk of blood clotting problems and HRT?

It is accepted that oral contraceptives in general and synthetic estrogens specifically are associated with an increased risk of blood clotting in brain, heart, lungs, and—most commonly—in the veins of the legs and pelvis. The increased risk of heart attack in women over the age of 35 and on birth control pills is well known. Despite these well-documented facts, *no* correlation has been found between the hormones used on hormone replacement therapy (HRT) and increased occurrence of blood clots.

The fact that most HRT uses estrogens derived from natural sources and that they are used in lower doses than found in birth control pills is considered to be the difference that avoids the blood-clotting problems.

All studies concerning use of progesterone have consistently shown no adverse effects on the clotting mechanism. If estrogen replacement therapy has been decided upon, cyclic progesterone therapy may be added without fear of inducing problems with blood clotting.

Women who have active blood-clotting problems such as thrombophlebitis or emboli should not start on hormone therapy until the active problem is resolved, and then they should proceed with caution. However, a woman who has simply experienced a thrombophlebitis that was not related to pregnancy, use of the Pill, or HRT has no reason to be denied HRT. Women who have had blood-clotting problems related to pregnancy or who use the Pill should be started on HRT with great caution and on lower doses of estrogen (Premarin, 0.625 milligram).

### Does HRT affect glucose metabolism?

There are conflicting reports about the effect of hormone replacement therapy (HRT) on metabolism of blood sugar (glucose). I have not found any increase in problems with blood sugars in my postmenopausal patients on HRT. Some symptomatic diabetic women may find that HRT worsens their diabetes. For the first three months, the physician should monitor the blood sugar levels of menopausal, diabetic women who start HRT.

Conclusive evidence shows that estrogen has no effect on glucose metabolism. The information is derived from studies on oral contraceptives, which use much higher doses of estrogen than does HRT.

Progesterone does have some adverse effect on glucose metabolism. Medroxyprogesterone (Provera) and norethindrone acetate (Agestin) seem to have only a small effect that is insignificant in healthy postmenopausal women.

## Does HRT harm the liver?

Rarely, women taking oral contraceptives develop a tumor of the liver. Thus far, these tumors have not been reported in women using estrogens in the menopause.

Estrogen does have effects on liver metabolism as described in the answer to the question "How does the potency of commercially available estrogen preparations compare?" (Chapter 5).

Therefore, women with previous histories of liver disease should be followed closely at the beginning of hormone replacement therapy (HRT). As noted, women with a history of jaundice (yellowing of the skin and the whites of the eyes) may get jaundice again during HRT. However, such recurrence of jaundice is rare.

Another rare condition, called "porphyria," can be triggered by various compounds including estrogen. One of the prominent symptoms of porphyria is acute abdominal pain. Women who have a diagnosis of porphyria should not use HRT.

## Under what conditions is HRT inadvisable?

The following list gives the conditions under which hormone replacement therapy (HRT) is inadvisable:
- Known or suspected cancer of the breast
- Known or suspected estrogen-dependent cancer
- Known or suspected pregnancy
- Undiagnosed abnormal vaginal bleeding
- Active thrombophlebitis or other problems with blood clotting
- History of blood-clotting disorders associated with previous estrogen use

Known or suspected cancer of the breast is thought to make HRT inadvisable because many of these breast cancers develop while the woman is still manufacturing her own estrogen. These tumors may be stimulated to grow in the presence of estrogen.

With the use of modern laboratory techniques, breast tumors are checked for estrogen receptor sites when they are removed. If the tumor contains significant numbers of estrogen receptor sites, then estrogen therapy should be avoided. However, if the tumor does not show significant estrogen receptor sites, it appears that estrogen therapy may be safe. Also recall that the use of progesterone reduces the number of estrogen receptor sites, especially when it has been used cyclically for at least four years. Perhaps future studies will show that cyclic estrogen-progesterone therapy is beneficial for women who have suffered from a breast cancer.

At present, most physicians treating women with breast cancer in which they lack information about estrogen receptor sites would suggest that the women avoid estrogen therapy. In my own practice, I have had several patients who have undergone radical surgery for breast cancer many years ago. They have been cautioned against estrogen therapy. With the development of menopausal symptoms that did not respond to nonhormonal therapies, the women reached a point where they felt the risk of HRT and the possible recurrence of their cancer was better than the intolerable, persistent symptoms of the postmenopause. Fortunately, I have not encountered any recurrence of cancer in these women who chose to use HRT.

Certain rare tumors are known to be estrogen-sensitive. Women afflicted with these tumors should avoid estrogen therapy.

The use of any drugs during pregnancy can endanger the fetus. Taking estrogen during pregnancy, especially during the first 12 weeks, increases the chance that the developing child will be born with a birth defect. The possiblity is small, however. In recent years there was a considerable amount of concern about the increased risk of female children developing cancer of the vagina or cervix during their teens or twenties, when the mother had ingested the drug DES. Since DES is a synthetic estrogen, the potential danger may also be present with use of other estrogen compounds, both synthetic and natural. (It should be noted that, to my knowledge, no medical conditions that occur in pregnancy would indicate the use of an estrogen compound.) Fortunately, pregnancy in the postmenopause is extremely rare.

With respect to undiagnosed abnormal bleeding, HRT is inadvisable only until the cause of bleeding has been properly diagnosed. This is because abnormal vaginal bleeding can be a sign of a uterine cancer. Use of HRT in the presence of abnormal vaginal bleeding caused by a uterine cancer might stop the bleeding and delay the diagnosis of the cancer. *If a woman who is to be started on menopausal HRT has had recent abnormal vaginal bleeding, she should have a physician evaluate the cause of the abnormal bleeding and reach a definitive diagnosis before she starts therapy.*

Blood-clotting disorders have already been discussed under the question "What about the risk of blood-clotting problems and HRT?" For these problems, the inadvisability of HRT applies only to those with *active* disease. The mere history of blood-clotting problems does not make HRT inadvisable. Only if the occurrence of these diseases was directly related to taking estrogen should the safety of HRT be questioned.

### Will HRT cause increased hair growth?

Increased hair growth is distasteful to most women. Many women do not realize that, as they enter the menopause, two changes within their bodies lead to increased hair growth.

Besides estrogen, all women produce some male hormone—testosterone. As a women approaches the menopause, her production of estrogen decreases, but the testosterone production remains the same. Since estrogen and testosterone basically neutralize each other, the decrease in estrogen results in a greater effect of testosterone. This relative increase in male hormone stimulates the hair follicles, thus increasing hair growth in women as they approach, and go through, the menopause.

The second change affecting hair growth in women as they approach the menopause is that the hair follicles themselves become more sensitive to testosterone and tend to accelerate their growth of hair. This is called increased "end organ" sensitivity.

These two changes mean that, to some extent, all women tend to have increased hair growth as they get older. As always, light-colored hair will be less noticeable and dark hair more noticeable.

Many years ago, before we fully understood how to use hormones properly, testosterone was given alone to stop hot flashes or was given along with the estrogen. The reason for this is that the testosterone suppressed estrogen's stimulation of the uterine lining. This suppression of growth in the uterine lining decreased or stopped uterine bleeding. If the estrogen was used without the testosterone, the women often developed undersirable vaginal bleeding. Although testosterone did suppress the uterine bleeding, it also had masculinizing effects on the woman. Most common was hair growth. But weight gain in the form of increased muscle mass, a lower voice, and a more masculine body shape also were problems in women receiving testosterone.

Thus, the use of HRT does not stimulate hair growth. Testosterone is not used in routine HRT.

### What about endometriosis and HRT?

Endometriosis is a disease in which the cells of the uterine lining are displaced into other areas of the body and grow there, cyclically. The most common area in which to find endometriosis growing is the pelvis. It has also been found on the cervix, in the umbilicus (belly button), and in the wall of the bowel.

As the ovary produces its cyclic hormones and stimulates the uterine lining to grow, the cells that have been displaced into other areas of the body are also stimulated to grow. When the ovarian hormone cycle ends each month, the uterine lining dies because of lack of progesterone. This causes the women to have a period. This same type of cell death and bleeding occurs in those displaced cells growing in other areas. The cells bleed into the surrounding tissues, causing small blisters of blood. The body then reacts to clean up the debris. This is known as an inflammatory reaction. This growth, death, bleeding, and inflammatory reaction in the misplaced cells and surrounding tissues causes pain before and during the menses. Pain with intercourse also is common. This whole process can lead to eventual scarring of the inflammed tissues, which can lead to infertility.

The cyclic hormones produced by the ovaries are really the cause of the problem. Endometriosis and all its symptoms are cured by the menopause, because all cyclic ovarian hormone production stops at that time. Hormone replacement therapy (HRT) causes the problems of endometriosis to continue in the menopause, since it attempts to reproduce the cyclic hormone production of the ovaries.

A woman who has symptomatic endometriosis during the premenopausal years should strongly consider surgical treatment of the endometriosis in the form of total abdominal hysterectomy and removal of the tubes and ovaries. This resolves the problems produced by the endometriosis long before the natural menopause. In addition, successful treatment of the endometriosis will allow the woman to use HRT in the postmenopausal period without recurrence of the aggravating symptoms of endometriosis.

One might ask, "If you take out the ovaries in order to stop stimulation of endometriosis, then why can you replace the hormones after surgery without causing the same symptoms?" Removing the uterus eliminates the main source of endometrial cells. Removal of the tubes, ovaries, and all visible endometriosis is intended to remove all the remaining disease. None is left to be stimulated. Even if some microscopic sites of endometrial cells are left behind, most will die during the six to eight weeks after surgery when the patient does not receive any hormones. When HRT begins, no endometrial cells are left to be stimulated.

In a few cases, this approach does not work as expected, and the endometriosis recurs. In those cases, hormone therapy can easily be withheld for longer periods of time in order to starve the remaining areas out of existence.

### What about uterine fibroids and HRT?

Uterine fibroids are dense growths of fibrous tissue on or within the uterus. They can be only an eighth of an inch in diameter, or they can reach diameters greater than a foot and weigh over 20 pounds.

Fibroids are found in many women during their childbearing years. Although rare, they can occur in young women in their 20s. They seem to become more prevalent in the 40s and 50s. Fewer than 1 percent become malignant. The most common symptoms of fibroids are irregular vaginal bleeding, heavy periods, pelvic pressure, and pelvic pain.

Unless a women is having symptoms from her fibroids or the fibroids are beginning to extend beyond the pelvis, there is no reason to remove them. Usually the physician will simply have the patient return for regular checkups every six to twelve months.

Hormones, especially estrogens, can stimulate fibroids to grow. Moreover, the size of the hormone dose seems to be related to the rate of fibroid growth. As a woman passes the age of 40 and her hormone production begins to vary, the growth of fibroids tends to be stimulated. As the woman enters the postmenopausal years with low estrogen levels, fibroids usually begin to get smaller. Many women, in trying to avoid hysterectomy, put up with aggravating symptoms caused by fibroids in hopes of reaching the menopause, when the symptoms will cease and the fibroids will decrease in size.

These women present a significant problem when it comes to hormone replacement therapy (HRT). On the one hand, they need and may want HRT to help them with their aggravating menopausal symptoms and to protect them from the degenerating changes that occur from estrogen deficiency. On the other hand, if they use HRT and replace the hormones up to the premenopausal level, the fibroids may again be stimulated to grow and cause symptoms. This is a serious dilemma.

A premenopausal woman who has a fibroid should elect to have a hysterectomy when the fibroid begins producing aggravating symptoms. Waiting for the menopause in hopes that the symptoms will subside and surgery will be avoided is illogical if the woman hopes to take advantage of hormone replacement therapy in the postmenopausal years. The advantages gained from using HRT in the postmenopause outweigh the discomfort and risk of the surgery.

The woman who reaches menopause with an asymptomatic fibroid should start the HRT just as if she had no fibroids. She should be followed with regular three-month checkups. If the fibroids start to grow or begin to produce aggravating symptoms, then a hysterectomy may be in order. The relatively short recovery period (six to eight weeks) required for surgery is worth the years of better health gained from using HRT in the postmenopausal years.

Many patients with fibroids at the time of menopause show no increase in fibroid growth or symptoms during the years of HRT.

## What about epilepsy and HRT?

Use of estrogen and/or progesterone can cause retention of fluid, and epilepsy can be aggravated by retention of fluid. In my experience, I have never seen postmenopausal epileptics have trouble with hormone replacement therapy (HRT). Even in female epileptics whom I have placed on birth control pills, with their larger doses of synthetic estrogens and their increased tendency to cause fluid retention, very few have had a related increase in seizures. However, as with any postmenopausal woman with a major disease, HRT should be initiated cautiously. The advantages of HRT usually outweigh the risks.

## Will I have to have periods all my life if I take HRT?

Women often think, "Thank goodness I won't have to put up with periods after I go through the menopause!" But remember, periods have always been the sign of a youthful woman; and if taking hormone replacement therapy (HRT) can help you keep your youthful health, they are worth the bother. Remember also that the monthly cyclic bleeding is decreasing your risk of uterine cancer.

In my experience, about 20 percent of the women taking cyclic hormones will stop having cyclic periods in their 60s. Most women using HRT will have stopped having periods by the age of 70. Of course, the women who have had a previous hysterectomy will not have any periods when using HRT.

Until now, women who have had their uterus surgically removed were treated with cyclic estrogen therapy only. They were not given cyclic progesterone on the basis that it was not needed if the uterus was absent. Today, however, evidence indicating a decrease in the rate of breast cancer with use of cyclic progesterone therapy suggests that even women without a uterus may want to include progesterone in their HRT.

Most of my postmenopausal patients state that the menstrual flow they have with HRT is shorter and lighter than their previous normal flow. But some patients are less fortunate and have heavy or long periods, painful periods, and sometimes a great deal of premenstrual tension syndrome. Various changes in the hormone preparations can sometimes alleviate these problems. It may even be necessary to treat the woman with additional medications for the premenstrual tension (see Appendix D). Again, the advantages gained from the HRT are well worth any bother you have to go through with additional medications.

# 7
# FINE-TUNING HORMONE REPLACEMENT THERAPY

*What can I do about heavy periods during HRT?*

Sometimes decreasing the dose of estrogen makes the periods lighter. However, doses of less than 0.625 milligram of conjugated estrogens are inadequate protection from osteoporosis. Switching the progesterone from Provera to one of the 19-nor-testosterones, such as Aygestin, may also cause the period to be lighter.

In rare cases, where a patient is about to give up hormone replacement therapy because of 12 uncomfortable periods a year, I suggest a 50-day cycle in order to cut the number of periods to six per year. Sometimes this convinces her to tolerate the periods. In this cycle, the woman takes estrogen for 50 days. The last 13 days she takes progesterone along with the estrogen. This longer progesterone therapy with 50-day estrogen cycles assures adequate emptying of the uterus with each period.

## What can I do for breast tenderness with HRT?

Usually a woman who starts HRT as soon as the menopause is reached will not notice any change in breast problems from what she had with her own periods. A woman who starts HRT after being in the postmenopause for some time will probably initially experience some breast fullness, enlargement, and/or tenderness soon after starting the HRT. Thankfully, in this latter group of women, the breast problems usually settle down or completely disappear within the first three months of therapy.

When the postmenopausal woman on HRT experiences these kinds of breast problems, she can do several things. First and foremost is to stop intake of all foods with caffeine and chocolate. (Chocolate contains the chemical xanthine, which has a similar effect on the breast as does caffeine.) I have been amazed at the number of women whose breast soreness has completely disappeared when they implemented this dietary change.

Diuretics reduce the amount of fluid in your body tissues, and they also can be helpful in treating these breast problems. These compounds must be used with caution, because they can deplete the body of potassium. Several products on the market are potassium-conserving and would be appropriate for this use. (Maxide and Dyazide are examples.) Oranges, bananas, and kiwi fruits are high in potassium; eating them is beneficial when using diuretics.

Decreasing the estrogen dose can also reduce breast problems. Remember, the estrogen dose should not be lowered below 0.625 milligram of conjugated estrogens for adequate protection against osteoporosis. In rare cases, switching to another estrogen preparation has helped decrease these breast problems.

### What can I do if I am on HRT but still have hot flashes?

This question has already been partially answered under the question "How do I know if my hormone dosage is correct?" (Chapter 5). Some women seem to have difficulty absorbing estrogen through the intestines. A physician can check this by giving a shot of a long-acting estrogen preparation to see whether the symptoms are alleviated.

Some women indicate that the hormone replacement therapy (HRT) they are using has helped most of their symptoms considerably, but they still are having some hot flashes. It seems that some women metabolize or excrete the estrogen taken orally more rapidly than other women. If they take their estrogen tablet in the morning, they are comfortable during the day, but by nighttime they are experiencing recurrent hot flashes. For these women, splitting their dosage of estrogen into a morning and an evening dose may take care of the problem. In fact, a few patients have had to take their estrogen in three doses during the day in order to alleviate all their hot flashes. In most of these cases, the total daily dose is the same; it is just spread out throughout the day.

Occasionally, relatively large doses are needed orally to get the desired effect. If one woman requires six times the dose of another woman in order to relieve her symptoms and if she does not experience any significant effects of overdosage, the higher doses should be used. That particular woman is simply breaking down and excreting the estrogen faster than the average woman. She is better off taking high oral doses than repeated shots of long-acting estrogens (see Appendix D).

## Can I do anything to avoid the menopausal symptoms I get on the days I am off my hormones each month?

Some women experience an immediate return of their hot flashes and depression during the few days each month that they are off their hormones. They often complain of headaches occurring during that time or just after they restart their hormone replacement therapy (HRT) each month. In these cases, the problem can be alleviated by giving the woman a daily dose of estrogen comparable to 0.3 milligram of conjugated estrogens for these few days at the end of each cycle.

Occasionally the dose may have to be as high as one half the daily dose of the HRT. On rare occasions, a woman requires the same dose of estrogen every day in order to remain comfortable. In those rare cases, I give her the same dose of estrogen every day, but she still takes the cyclic progesterone in the same way. These women have the usual menstrual flows seen in women who stop their estrogen when they complete the 10 days of progesterone, because it is not the cessation of the estrogen therapy that causes the menstrual flow, but rather the cessation of the progesterone.

# APPENDIX A
# FDA STATEMENTS

*What exactly do the FDA statements say about estrogens and increased risk of cancer?*

The following is a word-for-word copy of the statement of the FDA to physicians concerning estrogens.

**1. Estrogens have been reported to increase the risk of endometrial carcinoma.**

Three independent case control studies have reported an increased risk of endometrial cancer in postmenopausal women exposed to exogenous estrogens for more than one year. This risk was independent of the other known risk factors for endometrial cancer. These studies are further supported by the finding that incidence rates of endometrial cancer have increased sharply since 1969 in eight different areas of the United States with population-based cancer reporting systems, an increase which may be related to the rapidly expanding use of estrogens during the last decade. The three case control studies

111

reported that the risk of endometrial cancer in estrogen users was 4.5 to 13.9 times greater than in nonusers. The risk appears to depend on both duration of treatment and on estrogen dose. In view of these findings, when estrogens are used for the treatment of menopausal symptoms, the lowest dose that will control symptoms should be utilized and medication should be discontinued as soon as possible.

When prolonged treatment is medically indicated, the patient should be reassessed on at least a semiannual basis to determine the need for continued therapy. Although the evidence must be considered preliminary, one study suggests that cyclic administration of low doses of estrogen may carry less risk than continuous administration; it therefore appears prudent to utilize such a regimen. Close clinical surveillance of all women taking estrogens is important. In all cases of undiagnosed persistent or recurring abnormal vaginal bleeding, adequate diagnostic measures should be undertaken to rule out malignancy.

There is no evidence at present that 'natural' estrogens are more or less hazardous than 'synthetic' estrogens at equiestrogenic doses.

This is the exact warning that appears in a boxed enclosure in the *Physicians' Desk Reference*, 39th Edition, 1985, pages 664-667. It goes on to warn, "Estrogens should not be used during pregnancy." I agree with the statement regarding pregnancy.

In addition to this statement to physicians, the FDA has prepared a patient information statement. This must be given to the patient with each prescription for estrogen that is filled. That statement is as follows:

### INFORMATION FOR THE PATIENT

**What You Should Know About Estrogens:** Estrogens are female hormones produced by the ovaries. The ovaries make several different kinds of estrogens. In addition, scientists have been able to make a variety of synthetic estrogens. As far as we know, all these estrogens have similar properties and therefore much the same usefulness, side effects, and risks. This leaflet is intended to help you understand what estrogens are used for, the risks involved in their use, and how to use them as safely as possible.

This leaflet includes the most important information about estrogens, but not all the information. If you want to know more, you should ask you doctor for more information or you can ask your doctor or pharmacist to let you read the package insert prepared for the doctor. **Uses of Estrogen:** THERE IS NO PROPER USE OF ESTROGENS IN A PREGNANT WOMAN.

Estrogens are prescribed by doctors for a number of purposes including:

1. To provide estrogen during a period of adjustment when a woman's ovaries stop producing a majority of her estrogens, in order to prevent certain uncomfortable symptoms of estrogen deficiency. (With the menopause, which generally occurs between the ages of 45 and 55, women produce a much smaller amount of estrogens.)

2. To prevent symptoms of estrogen deficiency when a woman's ovaries have been removed surgically before the natural menopause.

3. To prevent pregnancy. (Estrogens are given along with a progestogen, another female hormone; these combinations are called oral contraceptives or birth control pills. Patient labeling is available to women taking oral contraceptives and they will not be discussed in this leaflet.)

4. To treat certain cancers in women and men.

5. To prevent painful swelling of the breasts after pregnancy in women who choose not to nurse their babies.

**Estrogens in the Menopause:** In the natural course of their lives, all women eventually experience a decrease in estrogen production. This usually occurs between ages 45 and 55 but may occur earlier or later. Sometimes the ovaries may need to be removed before natural menopause by an operation, producing a 'surgical menopause.'

When the amount of estrogen in the blood begins to decrease, many women may develop typical symptoms: feelings of warmth in the face, neck, and chest or sudden intense episodes of heat and sweating throughout the body (called 'hot flashes' or 'hot flushes'). These symptoms are sometimes very uncomfortable. Some women may also develop changes in the vagina (called 'atrophic vaginitis') which causes discomfort, especially during and after intercourse.

Estrogens can be prescribed to treat these symptoms of the menopause. It is estimated that considerably more than half of all women undergoing the menopause have only mild symptoms or no symptoms at all and therefore do not need estrogens. Other women may need estrogens for a few months, while their bodies adjust to lower estrogen levels. Sometimes the need will be for periods longer than six months. In an attempt to avoid overstimulation of the uterus (womb), estrogens are usually given cyclically during each month of use, such as three weeks of pills followed by one week without pills.

Sometimes women experience nervous symptoms or depression during menopause. There is no evidence that estrogens are effective for such symptoms without associated vasomotor symptoms. In the absence of vasomotor symptoms, estrogens should not be used to treat nervous symptoms, although other treatment may be needed.

You may have heard that taking estrogens for long periods (years) after the menopause will keep your skin soft and supple and keep you feeling young. There is no evidence that this is so, however, and such long-term treatment carries important risks.

**Estrogens to Prevent Swelling of the Breast After Pregnancy:** If you do not breast-feed your baby after delivery, your breasts may fill up with milk and become painful and engorged. This usually begins about 3 to 4 days after delivery and may last for a few days to up to a week or more. Sometimes the discomfort is severe, but usually it is not and can be controlled by pain-relieving drugs such as aspirin and by binding the breasts up tightly. Estrogens can be used to try to prevent the breasts from filling up. While this treatment is sometimes successful, in many cases the breasts fill up to some degree in spite of treatment. The dose of estrogens needed to prevent pain and swelling of the breasts is much larger than the dose needed to treat symptoms of the menopause and this may increase your chances of developing blood clots in the legs or lungs (see below). Therefore, it is important that you discuss the benefits and the risks of estrogen use with your doctor if you have decided not to breast-feed your baby.

**The Dangers of Estrogens:**

1. *Endometrial cancer.* There are reports that if estrogens are used in the postmenopausal period for more than a year, there is an increased risk of endometrial cancer (cancer of the lining of the uterus). Women taking estrogens have roughly 5 to 10 times as great a chance of getting this cancer as women who take no estrogens. To put this another way, while a postmenopausal woman not taking estrogens has 1 chance in 1,000 each year of getting endometrial cancer, a women taking estrogen has 5 to 10 chances in 1,000 each year. For this reason *it is important to take estrogens only when they are really needed.*

The risk of this cancer is greater the longer estrogens are used and when larger doses are taken. Therefore you should not take more estrogen than your doctor prescribes. *It is important to take the lowest dose of estrogen that will control symptoms and to take it only as long as it is needed.* If estrogens are needed for longer periods of time, your doctor will want to reevaluate your need for estrogens at least every six months.

Women using estrogens should report any vaginal bleeding to their doctors; such bleeding may be of no importance, but it can be an early warning of endometrial cancer. If you have undiagnosed vaginal bleeding, you should not use estrogens until a diagnosis is made and you are certain there is no endometrial cancer. *NOTE:* If you have had your uterus removed (total hysterectomy), there is no longer danger of developing endometrial cancer.

2. *Other possible cancers.* Estrogens can cause development of other tumors in animals, such as tumors of the breast, cervix, vagina, or liver, when given for a long time. At present there is no good evidence that women using estrogen in the menopause have an increased risk of such tumors, but there is no way yet to be sure they do not; and one study raises the possiblity that use of estrogens in the menopause may increase the risk of breast cancer many years later. This is a further reason to use estrogens only when clearly needed. While you are taking estrogens, it is important that you go to your doctor at least once a year for a physical examination. Also, if members of your family have had breast cancer or if you have breast nodules or abnormal mammograms (breast x-rays), your doctor may wish to carry out more frequent examinations of your breasts.

3. *Gallbladder disease.* Women who use estrogens after menopause are more likely to develop gallbladder disease needing surgery than women who do not use estrogens. Birth control pills have a similar effect.

4. *Abnormal blood clotting.* Oral contraceptives increase the risk of blood clotting in various parts of the body. This can result in a stroke (if the clot is in the brain), a heart attack (clot in a blood vessel of the heart), or a pulmonary embolus (a clot which forms in the legs or pelvis, then breaks off and travels to the lungs). Any of these can be fatal.

At this time use of estrogens in the menopause is not known to cause such blood clotting, but this has not been fully studied and there could still prove to be such a risk. It is recommended that if you have had clotting in the legs or lungs or a heart attack or stroke while you were using estrogens or birth control pills, you should not use estrogens (unless they are being used to treat cancer of the breast or prostate). If you have had a stroke or heart attack or if you have angina pectoris, estrogens should be used with great caution and only if clearly needed (for example, if you have severe symptoms of the menopause).

The larger doses of estrogen used to prevent swelling of the breasts after pregnancy have been reported to cause clotting in the legs and lungs.

**Special Warning About Pregnancy:** You should not receive estrogen if you are pregnant. If this should occur, there is a greater than usual chance that the developing child will be born with a birth defect, although the possibility remains fairly small. A female child may have an increased risk of developing cancer of the vagina or cervix later in life (in the teens or twenties). Every possible effort should be made to avoid exposure to estrogens during pregnancy. If exposure occurs, see your doctor.

**Other Effects of Estrogens:** In addition to the serious known risks of estrogens described above, estrogens have the following side effects and potential risks:

1. *Nausea and vomiting.* The most common side effect of estrogen therapy is nausea. Vomiting is less common.

2. *Effects on breasts.* Estrogens may cause breast tenderness or enlargement and may cause the breasts to secrete a liquid. These effects are not dangerous.

3. *Effects on the uterus.* Estrogens may cause benign fibroid tumors of the uterus to get larger.

4. *Effects on liver.* Women taking oral contraceptives develop, on rare occasions, a tumor of the liver which can rupture and bleed into the abdomen and may cause death. So far, these tumors have not been reported in women using estrogens in the menopause, but you should report any swelling or unusual pain or tenderness in the abdomen to your doctor immediately. Women with

a past history of jaundice (yellowing of the skin and white parts of the eyes) may get jaundice again during estrogen use. If this occurs, stop taking estrogens and see your doctor.

5. *Other effects.* Estrogens may cause excess fluid to be retained in the body. This may make some conditions worse, such as asthma, epilepsy, migraine, heart disease, or kidney disease.

**Summary:** Estrogens have important uses, but they have serious risks as well. You must decide, with your doctor, whether the risks are acceptable to you in view of the benefits of treatment. Except where your doctor has prescribed estrogens for use in special cases of cancer of the breast or prostate, you should not use estrogens if you have cancer of the breast or uterus, are pregnant, have undiagnosed abnormal vaginal bleeding, clotting in the legs or lungs or have had a stroke, heart attack or angina, or clotting in the legs or lungs in the past while you were taking estrogens.

You can use estrogens as safely as possible by understanding that your doctor will require regular physical examinations while you are taking them and will try to discontinue the drug as soon as possible and use the smallest dose possible. Be alert for signs of trouble including:

1. Abnormal bleeding for the vagina.

2. Pains in the calves or chest or sudden shortness of breath, or coughing blood.

3. Severe headache, dizziness, faintness, or changes in vision.

4. Breast lumps (you should ask your doctor how to examine your own breasts).

5. Jaundice (yellowing of the skin).


If you have read the preceding chapters you are aware that the above statement by the FDA contains passages which are no longer true, not adequately updated, and are misleading and erroneously threatening to the patient.

# APPENDIX B

# ADDITIONAL CAUSES OF HEAVY AND/OR PROLONGED MENSES

**FIBROID TUMORS OF THE UTERUS**

Fibrous growths of connective tissue on or within the wall of the uterus are called fibroids or leiomyomatas. Basically they are benign fibrous tumors. They range in size from a few millimeters to a foot or more in diameter. They represent the most common tumorous growth of the uterus.

The exact cause for these uterine fibrous growths is unknown. They occur more commonly in the middle and the latter half of the menstrual life. They seem to be definitely stimulated by estrogen, but estrogen itself does not seem to be their direct cause.

They usually can occur in three locations. They may appear on the surface of the uterus, causing the uterus to have an irregular shape. These types are called subserosal fibroids. They may have a broad base, or they may be on a pedicle, like a piece of fruit hanging from a branch. In most cases these types of fibroids do not cause much problem until they reach a large size. Then they can cause problems of pressure and simple crowding of other organs.

Fibroids that grow within the wall of the uterus are termed intramural fibroids. Usually they cause a symmetrical enlargement of the uterus. These fibroids cause the fewest symptoms. There may be many intramural fibroids, even large ones that distort the shape of the uterus and yet do not produce any symptoms. Fairly often, fibroids are found during a routine examination in a woman having no complaints related to the tumors.

Lastly are submucous fibroids. They are found growing into the uterine cavity. They distort the lining of the uterus and thin it out. This frequently causes excessive menstrual bleeding. Intramural fibroids, described earlier, can also become so large that they impinge upon the uterine cavity, distorting the lining and causing excessive menstrual bleeding. Both the submucous and intramural fibroids also distort the muscle fibers of the uterine wall, interfering with their normal contraction, which ordinarily helps to limit blood flow from the small uterine vessels during menses. The result can be excessive bleeding during menses. In addition, submucous fibroids can cause cramping. The uterus acts as if the submucous fibroid growing within the uterine cavity is a foreign body and tries to expel it by contracting. In some women, this causes severe cramps with periods.

In summary, fibroids, depending on their size and location, can cause excessive menstrual bleeding, pressure symptoms, and/or cramps.

### ENDOMETRIAL POLYPS

An excessive, localized outgrowth of uterine lining (endometrium) is called a polyp. These endometrial polyps may be single or multiple. They may hang down into the uterine cavity from a small pedicle, or they may be attached by a broad base. They vary in diameter from ¼ inch to 1½ inches. Although the mechanism is not clear, they can cause extremely heaving bleeding. If they hang by a long pedicle, they may also cause painful cramps as the uterus attempts to squeeze them out.

Endometrial polyps are more frequently found in the perimenopausal years. These polyps are most commonly benign, but they can be malignant. They are quickly and easily cured by scraping them out of the uterus by the procedures known as a dilatation and curettage (D&C).

## ADENOMYOSIS

When islands of uterine lining tissue are found scattered throughout the muscle of the uterine wall, the condition is called adenomyosis. Exactly how these endometrial lining cells get into the muscle is not known. One theory is that this is brought about by repeated pregnancies. Another is that they grow down into the muscle layers from the uterine cavity. Support for the first theory comes from the fact that adenomyosis is three to four times more common in women who have had several children than in women who have not had any children. As with fibroids and endometrial polyps, adenomyosis is found more frequently in women as they enter their 40s and 50s.

The study of uteri removed for all causes shows that 10 percent of these have adenomyosis. However, not all of the women complained of any symptoms. The most common two symptoms of this condition are painful and heavy periods. Mild enlargement of the uterus is also common.

The painful periods are probably caused by the actual bleeding of this endometrial tissue into the muscle while the woman is having her normal period. The endometrial cells are controlled by the hormones produced by the ovaries. Therefore, when the ovaries have completed their monthly cycle of hormone production, and the lining cells of the uterine cavity, which depend on these hormones for their growth, begin to die, the endometrial cells in the muscle of the uterus also begin to die and cause bleeding. This bleeding into the closed tissue space of the muscle cause the pain.

The cause of the heavy menstrual bleeding is unclear. It is probably related to the interference of the adenomyosis with the normal function of the uterine muscle. Control of uterine bleeding is different than for other types of bleeding. In uterine bleeding, the muscle fibers of the uterine wall contract around the blood vessels and squeeze them shut. Bleeding in other parts of the body is controlled by blood clotting.

The pain and heavy bleeding of adenomyosis are not alleviated by a D&C as with endometrial polyps. The only definitive cure for adenomyosis is hysterectomy. The only way to definitely diagnose adenomyosis is to examine the walls of the uterus microscopically after it has been removed. Therefore, adenomyosis is treated before it is diagnosed.

# APPENDIX C

# TERMINAL PROGESTERONE THERAPY (MEDICAL D&C)

As has been discussed, at various times during a woman's life she may have irregular uterine bleeding. After the age of 40, her physician must consider the possibility of a cancer of the uterus. In those cases, treatment with hormones to control the bleeding is inadvisable unless cancer has been ruled out. For women under 40, however, if lesions of the vagina and cervix have been ruled out, the cause of the bleeding is probably not a cancer and is most likely the result of an irregularity in hormone production.

These cases of irregular hormone production are called dysfunctional uterine bleeding. This condition is thought to occur either because an egg never developed for that cycle or because after ovulation a corpus luteum failed to develop or, if it did develop, produced inadequate amounts of progesterone.

As explained in the discussion of the menstrual cycle, estrogen is produced by the body of the ovary and, to a greater extent, by the developing egg. Estrogen causes the uterine lining to grow. However, it is the progesterone produced after ovulation by the corpus luteum that ripens the lining and causes the woman to have a concise period with complete shedding of the uterine lining. If an egg fails to develop during a cycle, it follows that ovulation and formation of a corpus luteum cannot occur during that cycle. If the corpus luteum never forms or if it functions inadequately in the second half of the menstrual cycle, then the uterine lining never ripens, and when a period does start, it will be abnormal. The period may be late, very heavy, erratic in flow, or prolonged with alternating flow and spotting.

A young woman with these symptoms and whose general physical and pelvic exams are otherwise normal has three alternatives as to therapy. First, she may simply choose to wait and hope for spontaneous improvement. If the bleeding is not so heavy that she is concerned about developing anemia, she has a 75 percent chance that it will resolve without therapy. This spontaneous cure occurs during the next cycle if she experiences a normal ovulation, formation of a corpus luteum, and adequate production of progesterone.

The second choice is to have a surgical D&C (dilatation and curettage). This is especially helpful in cases where the bleeding is extremely heavy and excessive blood loss is a concern. During a D&C, the lining is scraped out of the uterine cavity, and for all practical purposes the bleeding is stopped immediately.

The third alternative treatment is "terminal progesterone therapy." I use two forms of terminal progesterone therapy. The first is for women who are having a heavy and prolonged bleeding episode, when the main objective is to control them quickly. In these cases I prescribe a 21-pill pack of birth control pills containing strong doses of progesterone and estrogen. The patient takes five pills the first day, four the next, and three the next, two the next, and then one a day until all the pills are gone. This initial high dose of estrogen and progesterone causes the lining to stop degenerating. The estrogen in the pills causes the lining to start growing again, and the progesterone ripens the lining in preparation for the menses. Using the 21-pill pack in this manner, the woman will finish her pills in 11 days. By the time she finishes the pills, the lining has become ripened and is ready to make a clean slough. One or two days after she finishes the pills, a period should occur, cleaning out the uterine cavity. The patient is then allowed to continue without medication, and her normal cycles should return.

In women who are not having a heavy period at the time but are having recurrent heavy periods and/or irregular spotting, I usually use the second method of terminal progesterone therapy. In these cases I direct the patient to count 16 days from the first day of her period and then start taking an oral progestin such as Provera 10-milligram tablets or Aygestin 5-milligram tablets once a day for 10 days. Basically this gives the woman the needed progestin at the end of each cycle. This in turn should make her periods regular, shorter, lighter, and free from spotting. Many physicians have found this technique useful. It is commonly called a "medical D&C" because it cleans the lining out of the uterine cavity. I have already discussed this type of therapy for women who are having irregular periods just before the menopause, under the question "What about HRT for menstrual irregularities that occur just before the menopause?" (Chapter 5).

Some young women, 16 or older, have very irregular or infrequent periods. They may have always been this way, or they may have developed the condition. They may never have had a period. Women with this type of problem should be medically evaluated. Although serious tumors, temporary emotional problems, severe physical activity, or birth control pills can cause this problem, one of the most common causes is a condition known as polycystic or sclerocystic ovarian syndrome. When periods are infrequent or nonexistent, it is important to find the cause and treat it in order to establish regular menstrual cycles.

The uterine lining, which is stimulated to grow by the effect of estrogen, should be regularly ripened and sloughed out of the uterus. When it isn't, the risk of uterine cancer increases. Research has demonstrated that women who have polycystic ovarian syndrome with infrequent or no periods have a high incidence of uterine cancer early in life. Terminal progesterone therapy has been shown to stimulate regular periods in these women, thereby avoiding this increased rate of uterine cancer.

# APPENDIX D
# WHAT IS NEW AND IN THE FUTURE?

**THE NEW ESTROGEN SKIN PATCH**

The answer to the question "Is there more than one estrogen hormone?" (Chapter 5) discussed various commercially available estrogens. That discussion mentioned that the only available routes of administration of estrogen are pills and shots. In late 1986, CIBA pharmaceutical company began marketing a new transdermal (through the skin) method for the administration of estrogen in the form of estradiol. The product is called Estraderm and has become nicknamed the "estrogen patch."

Basically, it is a small round patch of clear plastic-like material in layers. Between the layers is a small quantity of liquid containing the estradiol. Around the edge of the patch is a ring of adhesive, which allows the patch to stick to the skin. The layer of plastic-like material in contact with the skin (the control membrane) releases the estradiol onto the skin at a controlled rate. The skin can absorb the estradiol into the bloodstream without having to change it chemically, as is necessary when estradiol is taken in pill form.

The estradiol in the patch is used up about every four days, so the user changes the patch twice a week. There are two different doses of patches, 0.05 and 0.10 milligram. The dose is varied by the size of the control membrane in contact with the skin. The low-dose patch has half as much area in contact with the skin—less than the area of a matchbook—as the higher dose patch.

One benefit of the Estraderm patch is that the skin absorbs the estradiol rapidly and efficiently, with little of the hormone converted to other forms of estrogen. Because the skin absorbs estrogen so much more efficiently, the 0.10-milligram patch produces approximately the same blood level of estradiol in a woman as 2 milligrams of estradiol taken orally. It also gives more constant blood levels of estrogen than result from taking pills or shots.

Another benefit of administering estrogen with a transdermal patch is that when the patch is removed, the blood level of estradiol declines rapidly. Blood levels of estrone and estradiol return to their preapplication levels within 24 hours after the patch is removed. This could be an advantage for the cyclic regimen of estrogen-progesterone described earlier. In the case of the orally administered estrogens, the estrone and estradiol take seven days or more to return to preapplication levels. Whether this delay in clearing the estrogen from the blood stream is of any significance as far as the woman's health is concerned, is not known at this time.

The final benefit of the transdermal patch is that, with the estradiol entering the bloodstream as estradiol rather than estrone, the liver does not have to process the estradiol. When estrogen is administered orally, it goes directly to the liver in the form of estrone. The liver then is stimulated to convert it into various estrogen forms. This stimulation of the liver also significantly stimulates other processes in the liver, which leads to production of various substances. These substances are, at times, thought to produce unwanted side effects such as weight gain, high blood pressure, and overstimulation of the liver. Because the transdermal route bypasses the liver and produces lower but more chemically active estrogen levels, the stimulation of the liver is minimal. The advocates of the transdermal route feel that this is a great advantage. But therein lies what I feel is the big disadvantage of the transdermal route.

One of the advantages of estrogen replacement therapy, as discussed in the question "How can women avoid cardiovascular hardening of the arteries?" (Chapter 3), is that it causes an advantageous change in the lipoproteins found in the blood, which helps suppress the development of atherosclerosis in postmenopausal women. The transdermal route does not provide this benefit. The available studies show this protection against atherosclerosis to be a significant improvement in the health of the postmenopausal woman. At the same time, the effects of oral estrogens on liver metabolism and thereby high blood pressure and/or weight are minimal in the majority of patients. Also, the value of the protective effects against atherosclerosis far outweigh the effects of stimulating the liver metabolism.

As already described, when any estrogen compound is taken orally, the intestine must first convert the estrogen into estrone sulfate before it can pass through the intestinal wall into the bloodstream. When it enters the bloodstream as estrone sulfate, it then has to be converted back to estradiol before the body can use it. Oral administration of estrogen leads to a ratio of estrone to estradiol that is not found naturally with the estrone blood levels being elevated. As seen in the following table, the Estraderm patch also leads to a ratio of estrone to estradiol not found naturally. But this ratio is in the opposite direction, with the estradiol being high. No one knows whether these nonphysiologic ratios, in either direction, are significant.

| Condition | Estrone/Estradiol Ratio |
|-----------|:-----------------------:|
| Premenopausal woman | 1:1 |
| Postmenopausal woman | 2-4:1 |
| Oral estrogen therapy | 3-6:1 |
| Dermal patch therapy | 1:2.5-9 |

A few additional points about Estraderm: It does relieve the symptoms of menopause at least as well as the oral estrogens. The onset of relief is rapid (about four hours). Estraderm has no side effects in the stomach or digestive system. Blood pressure does not increase. Although it does not improve the blood lipids in favor of protecting against atherosclerosis, it does not have adverse effects on lipids. There are few side effects. The patch is transparent, is not unattractive, and is comfortable to wear. It holds fast to skin even during bathing or swimming most of the time. It can be used with cyclic progesterone (an important consideration). Skin irritation is limited, and significant skin reactions seldom occur. Its twice-weekly application makes it simple to use, so patients may prefer this method.

Some women seem to be unable to absorb adequate levels of estrogen taken in pills. These women continue to have the symptoms of menopause even when taking estrogen. Others are unable to tolerate the oral estrogen because it causes stomach irritation. Some patients find that oral estrogens do not relieve their symptom of insomnia. Finally, in some women, oral estrogen excessively stimulates the liver, causing high blood pressure or abnormal liver function. For these patients, Estraderm may be the therapy of choice.

The Estraderm transdermal system is a significant hormonal treatment of the menopausal female. But for the time being, except in special cases, the oral route of administration, with its additional protective effects against atherosclerosis, is still the method of choice for HRT.

**ESTROGEN DEFICIENCY AND ALZHEIMER'S DISEASE**
At a recent annual meeting of the Society of Neuroscience, Dr. Howard Fillit of the Rockefeller University laboratory of neuroendocrinology, New York, presented findings indicating that postmenopausal estrogen deficiency may play a role in the development of Alzheimer's disease. In a small group of elderly women with Alzheimer's, he found that their serum estrogen levels were significantly lower than in women with benign senile memory loss or in elderly women with no memory loss. It is not apparent from his studies whether this low estrogen level results from the hormone changes that occur in Alzheimer's or actually contributes to the progression of the disease.

Dr. Fillit and his colleagues are engaged in additional studies to see the effect of estrogen replacement therapy (ERT) on Alzheimer's disease. Initial results suggest that ERT has improved cognitive function in approximately one-third of the patients treated. The patients with milder symptoms seem to respond better than those with more severe symptoms. The results of these studies may prove helpful for women suffering from Alzheimer's.

## CIGARETTE SMOKING
## AND POSTMENOPAUSAL WOMEN

Cigarette smoking is one of the major health problems for women in the United States. Lung cancer has finally surpassed breast cancer to become the leading cancer killer of women. Smoking greatly increases the risk of arteriosclerotic heart disease.

A 1985 article in the *New England Journal of Medicine* indicates that women who smoke have lower levels of serum estrogen whether they are on HRT or not. Further, they have less protection against osteoporosis, have thinner bones, and enter the menopause at an earlier age. No intelligent person can doubt that *cigarette smoking is a major health hazard.*

**PREMENSTRUAL TENSION SYNDROME (PMS)**

PMS is said to affect 40 percent of menstruating women to varying degrees. We do not understand the biochemical cause of PMS. Oral contraceptives seem to decrease its occurence. Elimination of caffeine and chocolate from a woman's diet, ingestion of extra vitamin B6 (100 milligrams per day), and occasional use of a diuretic seem to help.

When a woman reaches the menopause and stops having periods, PMS no longer occurs. Unfortunately, in a small percentage of women who use HRT in the menopause, PMS symptoms may resume. PMS does not occur in those few postmenopausal women who use estrogen only. It seems to be a problem only in women who also use the progestin therapy. This is not surprising, since younger women experience the symptoms of PMS only in the last half of their cycle, when their ovaries are producing progesterone. These facts point to progesterone as the culprit.

In that small percentage of postmenopausal women on HRT who experience PMS, three methods are available for handling the problem. The least acceptable choice is to stop using the progestin altogether. This leaves the woman vulnerable to irregular and heavy menses or, worse yet, increased risk of uterine cancer as described in the question "What about hormones and uterine cancer?" (Chapter 4). This method is only a last resort.

Changing the progestin sometimes helps. If the woman is using Provera, a change to Aygestin may alleviate the problem.

The third and most effective method is the use of natural progesterone vaginal capsules. This method has proved successful in young premenopausal women with PMS. The capsules are not commercially manufactured by any one of the large pharmaceutical houses in the United States. The physician must have the local pharmacist make them up. The dosage of progesterone may vary fom

50 to 400 milligrams per capsule. Usually the patient inserts the dose found effective for her into the vagina each evening starting 2-14 days before her period, depending upon when she usually starts experiencing symptoms of PMS.

In postmenopausal patients on HRT who are experiencing significant PMS, these vaginal capsules have provided effective relief. The postmenopausal woman uses the progesterone vaginal capsules in place of the tablets she had been using for the last 10-14 days of her 25-day cycle of estrogen. I usually start with a 200-milligram daily dose. If this is effective, I then decrease the dose each month until I find the lowest dose that is still effective. Only rarely do I have to use a dose higher than 200 milligrams.

## HRT AND RHEUMATOID ARTHRITIS

In recent years there have been a number of studies which have shown evidence of a protective effect against the development of rheumatoid arthritis in women who have used oral contraceptives. The initial study done by the Royal College of General Practitioners in Great Britain showed as much as a 50% decrease in the development of rheumatoid arthritis among young women who used oral contraceptives. This early study has been confirmed by large studies in Sweden and the Netherlands.

A recent study carried out in the Netherlands and published in the March 1986 *Journal of the American Medical Association* indicates that the use of noncontraceptive hormones in perimenopausal and postmenopausal women (estrogen replacement therapy) decreased the incidence of development of rheumatoid arthritis in those women. This study goes along with the Great Britain findings.

It is too early to accept these findings as proven facts, since there are some studies which do not confirm them. However, it is my personal feeling that in the final analysis it will be shown that HRT does indeed decrease the development of rheumatoid arthritis in peri- and postmenopausal women.

It should be noted that while HRT may decrease the incidence of development of rheumatoid arthritis there is no evidence that use of HRT helps rheumatoid arthritis that is already present.

# SUMMARY

The woman of today is much different from the woman of the past. Because of better medicines, better foods, and better living conditions, a woman who has reached 50 can now expect to live, on an average, to the age of 85. This means she will live at least 37 years longer than she would have in 1900. It also means that more women will be in the menopause longer than ever before. Most of today's women will spend at least a third of their lives in the menopause. These facts have made the menopause a new deficiency disease.

All of a woman's life, her body has had, used, and depended on estrogen. When a woman enters the post-menopausal period of her life, she becomes estrogen-deficient. She then experiences withdrawal effects in the form of hot flashes, irritability, depression, lethargy, fatigue, and forgetfulness. If she waits and tolerates these symptoms long enough, most of them will subside—or at least she will learn to accept and live with them.

However, at the same time that she is experiencing these subjective symptoms, many of her organs and body systems are degenerating from lack of estrogen. The bones lose calcium and some of their basic supportive structure. In some women this occurs rapidly; in others, more slowly. The skin, bladder lining, and vaginal lining become thinner. This leads to irritated, dry skin; urinary burning and frequency; and a weakened vagina susceptible to infection, bleeding, and painful intercourse.

The low rate of cardiovascular disease enjoyed by premenopausal women disappears as the lack of estrogen allows faster atherosclerosis of the blood vessels. Within 10 to 15 years of being in the menopause, women, who previously had less chance of having a heart attack than men of the same age, now have almost the same chance of having a heart attack than their male counterparts.

Whereas cancer of the lining of the uterus is virtually unheard of in the normal menstruating woman, it begins to appear with increasing frequency after the menopause. This results from a combination of individual susceptibility, production of smaller quantities of estrogen, and lack of cyclic progesterone to protect the uterine lining from becoming cancerous.

Finally, although not positively proven yet, loss of progesterone production seems to be related to the increasing rate of breast cancer in the aging woman.

*All of these symptoms and changes are either totally stopped, reversed, or significantly slowed down through the use of cyclic estrogen-progesterone hormone replacement therapy (HRT).*

Clearly, the benefits of HRT far outweigh the possible risks. Further, the inconveniences of HRT, such as the need to take the pills daily, the possible aggravating but mild side effects of the hormones, and the possibility of having periods into the late 60s, are definitely worth the benefits. For various reasons, not all women can, or should, take HRT, but at least 90 percent of today's women can if they so desire. All women who reach the menopause should strongly consider hormonal replacement therapy.

# INDEX